Rad Tech's Guide to Photon Counting Computed Tomography

Euclid Seeram, PhD., FCAMRT

Adjunct Associate Professor; Medical Imaging and Radiation Sciences; Monash University, Clayton, Victoria, Australia

Adjunct Professor; Medical Radiation Sciences, Faculty of Health, University of Canberra, Bruce, Australian Capital Territory, Australia

Regular Guest Lecturer; Vision, Compassion, Awareness (VCA) Education Solutions for Health Professionals Inc., Toronto, Ontario, Canada

WILEY

Dedication

This book is dedicated to my smart and caring son, Dave, the best Dad on the planet, with love and blessings forever.

Contents

Preface

Photon Counting Computed Tomography (PCCT) has been hailed as one of two "monumental" developments in Computed Tomography (CT) by the National Institute of Biomedical Imaging and Bioengineering (NIBIB). The other is using Artificial Intelligence to improve brain CT imaging. Both have been cleared for clinical use by the Food and Drug Administration (FDA). PCCT is expected to become the new generation of X-ray CT. This book is about PCCT imaging systems.

The major characteristic of PCCT is that of the detector. While conventional CT systems use Energy Integrating Detectors (EIDs) based on Scintillators such as Gadolinium Oxysulfide (Gd_2O^2S) or Cadmium Tungstate ($CdWO_4$) to convert X-ray photons to light photons, which are then subsequently converted to electrical signals that are digitized and sent to the computer for processing; the PCCT detector is a Photon Counting Detector (PCD) based on the use of semiconductors such as Cadmium Telluride (CdTe) or Cadmium Zinc Telluride (CZT). PCDs convert X-ray photons directly to electrical signals that are digitized and sent to the computer for processing.

By virtue of their design, PCDs offer several advantages compared with EID CT imaging systems, namely, reduction of electronic noise, improved spatial resolution, improved contrast and contrast-to-noise ratio (CNR) reduced radiation dose, reduction of image artifacts, and material specific imaging. For example, the advantage of the absence of electronic noise and greater dose efficiency has been shown to decrease the radiation dose of whole-body low-dose CT examinations by over 50%. Furthermore, these advantages have provided gains in the clinical applications of PCCT to image small lesions, visualize microstructures, measure iodine concentrations, and reduce radiation dose, thus demonstrating that PCCT is a "valuable tool for disease diagnosis, treatment planning, and monitoring in various medical scenarios" (Ref. 17 in Chapter 6).

The major purpose of this book, *Rad Tech's Guide to Photon Counting Computed Tomography*, is to provide a useful resource to meet the developing educational requirements of the imaging personnel, not only in the United States and Canada, but also in the United Kingdom, Continental Europe, South America, Africa, Asia, and Australia and New Zealand.

The contents in this book are organized into 6 Chapters as follows:

Chapter 1 provides a brief description of CT, as presented by the pioneers Godfrey Hounsfield and Allan Cormack. Second, three major processes involved in CT imaging, namely Data Acquisition, Image Reconstruction, and Image Display and Communications, are reviewed, followed by a short overview of the evolution of CT detectors, leading to the introduction of photon counting detectors, used in current state-of-the-art CT scanners.

Chapter 2 presents a review of the essential physics of radiation attenuation in CT, followed by a description of the physical principles of MSCT imaging, including a review of CT image quality, in an effort to set the stage for understanding current state-of-the-art CT technology, photon counting CT.

Chapter 3 presents a comprehensive description of the fundamental physical principles of PCCT, including the technical design characteristics of their semiconductor sensors and associated electronics. Finally, the advantages of PCDs compared to EIDs are identified.

Chapter 4 outlines the advantages (listed above) of PCCT systems compared with CT systems using EIDs. Second, each advantage is illustrated with selected anatomical areas.

Chapter 5's objective is threefold: (i) to provide a general overview of QC with respect to definitions, followed by a brief description of three fundamental steps of QC; (ii) to summarize the elements of the ACR manual for QC of CT systems; and (iii) to outline key findings of a major study on establishing a quality assurance program for a PCD CT imaging system.

Chapter 6 provides an overview of the clinical applications of PCCT.

Enjoy, study, and learn from the pages that follow and remember – your patients will benefit from your wisdom.

Euclid Seeram, PhD
British Columbia, Canada

Acknowledgments

An important satisfying task in writing a book of this nature is to thank those medical physicists, biomedical engineers, computer scientists, radiologists, and manufacturers who have done the original work on the various topics included in this book.

In particular, I acknowledge Dr Liqiang Ren, Dr Bin Zheng, and Dr Hong Liu of the Center for Biomedical Engineering and School of Electrical and Computer Engineering, University of Oklahoma, Norman, OK, USA, whose tutorial on *X-ray Photon Counting Detector* provided me with the knowledge of not only the physics of PCD CT imaging, but also the essential technology of PCDs. Thank you all for what I personally consider the most comprehensive tutorial from which I have gained a useful insight into PCD CT imaging systems.

Additionally, I am grateful to several other individuals (*and their coauthors*) whose published works have enhanced my understanding of the nature of PCCT, including the physics and technology of photon counting detectors, as well as the clinical applications of PCD CT imaging: They are, in alphabetical order: *Dr Zaki Ahmed* of the Department of Radiology, Mayo Clinic, Rochester, MN; *Dr Mats Danielsson,* Department of Physics, KTH Royal Institute of Technology, AlbaNova University Center, and Prismatic Sensors AB, AlbaNova University Center, Stockholm, Sweden, whose work was published in *Physics in Medicine and Biology*; *Dr Thomas Flohr* of Siemens Healthcare GmbH, Computed Tomography, Forchheim, German, whose work was published in *Physica Medica*; *Dr Shuai Leng* and *Dr Cynthia McCollough*, both from the Department of Radiology, Mayo Clinic, Rochester, MN; *Dr Yuko Nakamura*, Diagnostic Radiology, Hiroshima University, Hiroshima, Japan, whose work was published in the *Japanese Journal of Radiology*; and *Dr Yingyi Wu* from the Department of Radiology, West China Hospital, Sichuan University, Chengdu China.

Furthermore, I am indebted to Julie Hinds, Director of Communications and Pam Halvaei, Traffic and Production Coordinator, American Society of Radiologic Technologists, for permission to use materials from two of my published articles in the *ASRT Journal* (see Chapters 2 and 3 for these references).

I am also grateful to all the anonymized reviewers of the proposal for this book. Thanks for your constructive comments and positive feedback on the need for this book.

Another individual to whom I owe a good deal of thanks is Valentina Al Hamouche, MRT(R), MSc, who is the CEO/Founder VCA Education Solutions for Health Professionals based in Toronto, Canada. Valentina has provided me with recurring opportunities to provide Radiographic Imaging Sciences and CT Physics and Technology and other topics such as *AI in Medical Imaging* delivered through live webinars to further educate technologists and students across Canada and internationally as well. Thank you, Valentina.

I am sincerely thankful to Tom Marriott, Senior Commissioning Editor: Nursing, Midwifery, and Allied Health at Wiley in the UK, for his speed and efficiency in getting me a contract and for his support throughout the process. Thanks to Christabel Daniel Raj, Managing Editor, Health Professions & Vet Medicine at Wiley, Chennai, India, whose work in the production process is much appreciated. Furthermore, I acknowledge the assistance of two other individuals from Wiley, namely Angelica Day, Editorial Assistant, Health Sciences, London, UK; and Anjali Godiyal (Ms), Permissions Specialist, Content Operations, Learning.

Last but certainly not least, I humbly acknowledge the support from my loving and beautiful family; first, my lovely wife, Trish, a warm, smart, caring, and a very special person in my life, thank you, Babes. Second, my caring and very brilliant son David, the best Dad on the planet, to his two most precious daughters, my granddaughters. Thanks for your enduring love, support, and encouragement.

Euclid Seeram, PhD
British Columbia, Canada

1

The Invention of the Computed Tomography Scanner and the Nobel Prize

Chapter at a Glance

Rad Tech's Guide to Photon Counting Computed Tomography,
First Edition. Euclid Seeram.
© 2025 John Wiley & Sons, Inc. Published 2025 by John Wiley & Sons, Inc.

Introduction

Computed tomography (CT) is a sectional imaging modality that has been used for several decades as a diagnostic tool in medicine. CT is based on tomographic principles to collect attenuation data from the patient and subjecting these data to complex computer software referred to as image reconstruction algorithms to create sectional anatomical slices of the patient through computer processing.

The purpose of this chapter is to outline in a comprehensive manner a brief description of CT as presented by the pioneers of this imaging modality, identify three major processes involved in CT imaging, and identify the fundamental elements of the evolution of CT detectors leading to the introduction of photon-counting detectors used in current state-of-the-art CT scanners.

What Is Computed Tomography?

The 1979 Nobel Prize in Physiology or Medicine was awarded to Godfrey N. Hounsfield and Allan M. Cormack "for the development of computer assisted tomography" [1]. In his Nobel Prize lecture, Hounsfield stated that "Computed Tomography ... measures the attenuation of X-ray beams passing through sections of the body from hundreds of different angles, and then, from the evidence of these measurements, a computer is able to reconstruct pictures of the body's interior ... based on the separate examination of a series of contiguous cross sections, as though we looked at the body separated into a series of thin "slices" [2].

Invention of the Computed Tomography Scanner: Contribution of the Pioneers

CT was invented in the 1970s as a diagnostic tool for the noninvasive clinical examination of the human brain [3–5].

This development was championed by two notable individuals, namely, Godfrey Newbold Hounsfield and Allan Cormack [6].

Godfrey Newbold Hounsfield

The literature includes numerous articles on Hounsfield and Cormack. This section will summarize the major contributions of each of them. Hounsfield was born in 1919 in Nottinghamshire, England. After his studies in electronics and electrical and mechanical engineering, he joined the staff at Electronic and Musical Industry (EMI Limited) in 1951 and began working on radar systems and later on computer technology.

In 1967, Hounsfield was investigating pattern recognition and reconstruction techniques by using the computer. During his research, he subsequently deduced that, passing an X-ray beam through an object at different angles, recording X-ray transmission readings, and processing these measurements would provide information about the internal structures of that object. His initial experiments used radiation from an americium gamma source coupled with a sodium iodide crystal detector, and it took about 9 days to scan the object. The computer needed 2.5 hours to process the 28,000 measurements collected by the detector. Since this procedure was too long, the gamma radiation source was replaced by a diagnostic X-ray tube. The results of these experiments were more accurate and took 1 day to produce a picture [5].

In 1971, the first clinical prototype CT brain scanner (EMI Mark 1) was installed at Atkinson-Morley's Hospital and clinical studies were conducted under the direction of Dr. Ambrose. The processing time for the picture was reduced to about 20 minutes. Later, with the introduction of minicomputers, the processing time was reduced further to 4.5 minutes [5]. In 1972, Hounsfield received the McRobert Award and subsequently earned several prestigious awards such as a Fellowship of the Royal Society and the Lasker Prize in the United States. In 1977, Hounsfield was appointed Commander of the British Empire, and in 1979, he shared the Nobel Prize in physiology or medicine with Allan MacLeod Cormack, a physics professor at Tufts University in Medford, Massachusetts, for their contributions to the development of CT. After receiving this prestigious prize, he was knighted by her majesty Queen Elizabeth II and became an Honorary Fellow of the Royal Academy of Engineering. Sir Godfrey Hounsfield died on August 12, 2004, at age 84 [6]. Additional details of Hounsfield's pioneering work can be found in a book titled *Godfrey Hounsfield: Intuitive Genius of CT* by Bates et al. [7], who were friends of Hounsfield and worked with him at EMI.

Allan MacLeod Cormack

Allan MacLeod Cormack was born in Johannesburg, South Africa, in 1924. He attended the University of Cape Town, where he obtained a bachelor of science in physics in 1944 and earned a master of science in crystallography in 1945. In 1958, he joined the physics department at Tufts University in the United States.

Professor Cormack developed solutions to the mathematical problems in CT. It was not until Hounsfield began work on the development of the first clinically useful CT scanner that Cormack's work addressed the solution to the mathematical problem in CT [8]. Cormack died at age 74 in Massachusetts on May 7, 1998. Furthermore, Professor Cormacposthumously received the Order of Mapungubwe, South Africa's highest honor, in December 2002, for his contribution to the invention of the CT scanner. On October 1, 2021, CT imaging completed 50 years of being a diagnostic tool in medicine [9].

Physical Principles and Technology of Computed Tomography: A Brief Overview

From the description of CT imaging by Hounsfield in the previous section, and noting that Cormack worked out the solutions to the mathematical problem in CT, it is useful to describe the fundamental elements in the CT imaging process, as a means of laying the foundation for Chapter 2.

Major Processes of Computed Tomography Imaging

The fundamental principles of CT imaging have been described in several textbooks on CT [10–12], and each has identified three major processes: data acquisition, image reconstruction, and image display, storage, and communications, as illustrated in Figure 1.1. The data acquisition system components are shown in Figure 1.2 and include the X-ray tube, detectors, and detector electronics. The purpose of the data acquisition system is not only to produce an X-ray beam from the X-ray tube, but also to measure the initial intensity of the beam from the X-ray tube and the intensity of the X-ray beam passing through the patient. The detector electronics

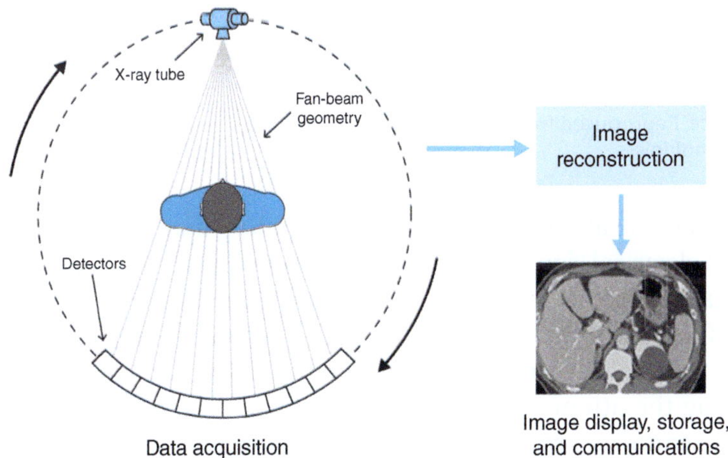

Figure 1.1 Three major processes used by a conventional computed tomography scanner to produce diagnostic-quality images.

Source: Reproduced from Seeram [13]/American Society of Radiologic Technologists.

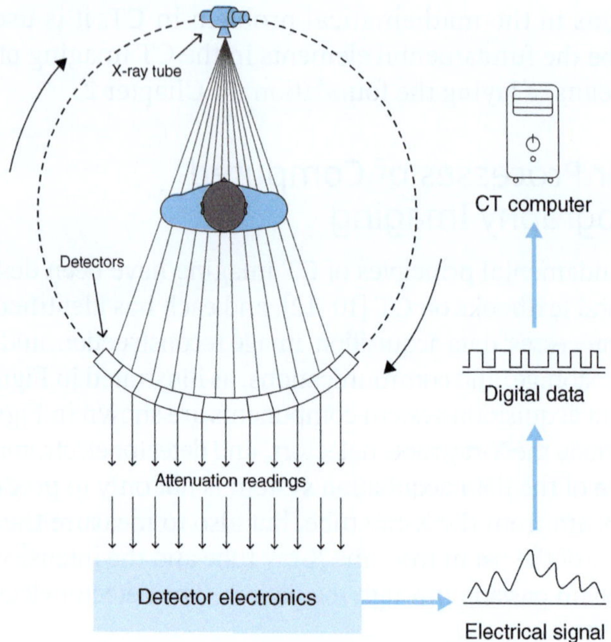

Figure 1.2 The major system components of the data acquisition system, illustrating the X-ray tube, the detectors, and the detector electronics.

Source: Reproduced from Seeram [13]/American Society of Radiologic Technologists.

convert the attenuated X-ray photons falling upon the detectors into electrical signals that are subsequently converted into digital data for processing by a mid-range computer system.

The next major process is image reconstruction. In this step, complex computer algorithms are used to create images using the attenuation data collected from the patient during the scanning process. The algorithms provide the solution to the mathematical problem in CT and have evolved through the years, from the filtered back projection and iterative recon-struction algorithms to reconstruction algorithms based on artificial intelligence (AI) [14]. While the older algorithms resulted in both poor image quality in low-dose CT imaging and long reconstruction times, AI-based algorithms have demonstrated improved image quality, especially in low-dose CT imaging [15–17].

A more detailed description of these algorithms will be reviewed in Chapter 2.

The final process deals with image display, storage, and communications. In this step, images are viewed on a monitor for interpretation, stored using appropriate storage devices, and subsequently distributed using a Medical Image Management and Processing System (MIMPS), formerly referred to as Picture Archiving and Communication System (PACS) [18].

The Evolution of Computed Tomography Detectors

Since this book deals with a new detector system referred to as a photon-counting detector, a brief review of the evolution of detectors used in CT is warranted. The detector used by Hounsfield when he invented the CT scanner (EMI Mark-4) [5] was a *solid-state scintillation detector* that used sodium iodide crystals coupled to a photomultiplier (PM) tube. Other scintillators such as calcium fluoride, bismuth germanate, cadmium tungstate, and cesium iodide were used as well [5]. While the scintillator converts X-ray photons into light photons, the PM tube converts the light photons into electrical signals. These detectors have been referred to as *indirect conversion detectors*, that is, X-ray photons are first converted into light photons, which are then converted into electrical signals (analog signals). These analog signals are subsequently converted into digital data and input into a computer for processing.

The use of scintillation detectors, or indirect conversion detectors, continued for several years. Having been used in single detector row spiral/helical CT, these are currently used in multidetector row spiral/helical CT. These scanners have been referred to as *multislice CT (MSCT) scanners* [19]. These detectors will be described further in Chapter 2.

Photon-Counting Detectors: Current State of Computed Tomography Imaging

The evolution continued using indirect conversion detectors for decades until recently when the direct conversion detectors appeared (Figure 1.3). The first direct conversion detector used xenon gas to convert X-ray photons directly into electrical signals. Eventually, xenon detectors became obsolete since they did not prove to be efficient. The second direct conversion detector is now a major system component in photon-counting CT scanners (Figure 1.3). Photon-counting detectors use semiconductors such as cadmium telluride to directly convert incoming X-ray photons into electrical charges [20]. The fundamental differences between indirect and direct conversion detectors are illustrated

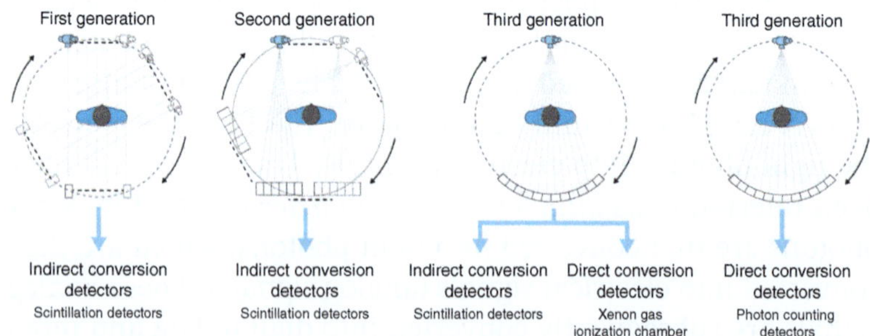

Figure 1.3 A generalized evolution of computed tomography detector types.

Source: Reproduced from Seeram [13]/American Society of Radiologic Technologists.

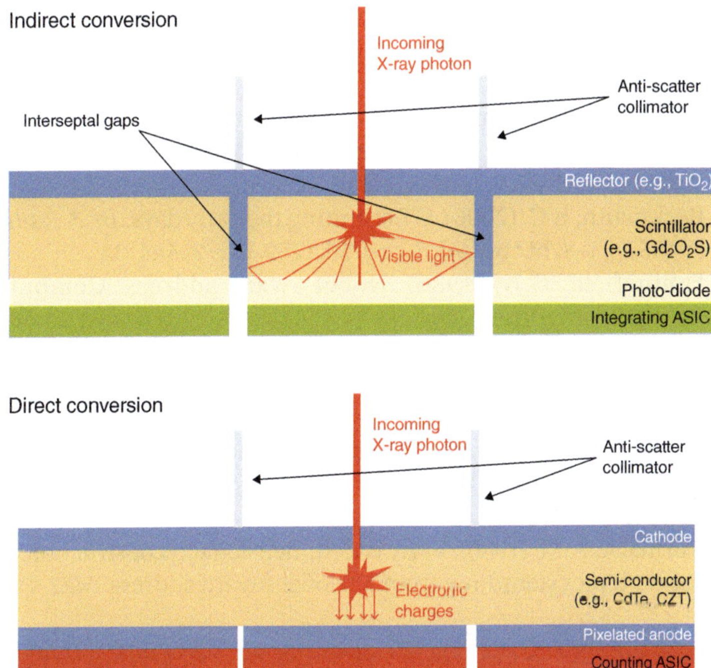

Figure 1.4 The fundamental differences between indirect and direct conversion detectors.

Source: Si-Mohamed et al. [20]/MDPI/CC BY 4.0.

in Figure 1.4. These evolutionary developments are intended to provide better spatial resolution and reduced image noise, especially in low-dose CT imaging.

The physical principles of photon-counting detectors will be described in detail in Chapter 3.

References

1 Godfrey, N. (2024). Hounsfield – facts. NobelPrize.org. Nobel Prize Outreach AB 2024. Tue. https://www.nobelprize.org/prizes/medicine/1979/hounsfield/facts/ (accessed 17 September 2024).

2 Hounsfield, G.N. (1980). Computed medical imaging, Nobel Award address. *Med. Phys.* 7: 283–290, 1980.

3 Bhattacharyya, K.B. (2016). Godfrey Newbold Hounsfield (1919-2004): the man who revolutionized neuroimaging. *Ann. Indian Acad. Neurol.* 19 (4): 448–450. https://doi.org/10.4103/0972-2327.194414.

4 Beckmann, E.C. (2006). CT scanning the early days. *Br. J. Radiol.* 79 (937): 5–8. https://doi.org/10.1259/bjr/29444122.

5 Hounsfield, G.N. (1980). Nobel award address. Computed medical imaging. *Med. Phys.* 7 (4): 283–290. https://doi.org/10.1118/1.594709.

6 Isherwood, I. (2004). Sir Godfrey Newbold Hounsfield–in memoriam. *Eur. Radiol.* 14: 2152–2153.

7 Bates, S., Beckman, L., Thomas, A., and Waltham, R. (2012). Godfrey Hounsfield: intuitive genius of CT. *Br. J. Radiol.* 85 (1019): e1165.

8 Cormack, A.M. (1980). Early two-dimensional reconstruction and recent topics stemming from it, Nobel Award address. *Med. Phys.* 7: 277–282.

9 McCollough, C. (2021). *Celebrating 50 Years of CT Imaging.* International Society for Computed Tomography.

10 Seeram, E. (2022). *Computed Tomography: Physical Principles, Patient Care, Clinical Applications, and Quality Control*, 5e. Maryland Heights, MO: Elsevier.

11 Bushberg, J.T., Seibert, A.J., Leidholdt, E.M. Jr., and Boone, J.M. (2021). *The Essential Physics of Medical Imaging*, 4e. Philadelphia, PA: Wolters Kluwer.

12 Kalender, W.A. (2011). *Computed Tomography: Fundamentals, System Technology, Image Quality, Applications*, 3e. Erlangen: Publicis Publishing.

13 Seeram, E. (2023). *Photon Counting Computed Tomography. Essential Education. CE Directed*, 1–13. Reading, MA: American Society of Radiologic Technologists (ASRT).

14 Zhang, Z. and Seeram, E. (2020). The use of artificial intelligence in computed tomography image reconstruction – a literature review. *J. Med. Imaging Radiat. Sci.* 51 (4): 671–677. https://doi.org/10.1016/j.jmir.2020.09.001.

15 Hsieh, J., Liu, E., Nett, B. et al. (2019). A new era of image reconstruction: TrueFidelity. https://www.gehealthcare.ru/jss media/040dd213fa894463287155151fdb01922.pdf (accessed September 2024).

16 Willemink, M.J. and Noël, P.B. (2019). The evolution of image reconstruction for CT-from filtered back projection to artificial intelligence. *Eur. Radiol.* 29 (5): 2185–2195. https://doi.org/10.1007/s00330-018-5810-7.

17 Boedeker, K. (2019). AiCE deep learning reconstruction: bringing the power of ultra-high resolution CT to routine imaging. *Canon Med. Syst.* 2: 28–33.

18 Medical Devices (2021). Medical device classification regulations to conform to medical software provisions in the 21st century cures act: a rule by the food and drug administration in 2021 (19 April 2021).

19 Booij, R., Budde, R.P.J., Dijkshoorn, M.L., and van Straten, M. (2020). Technological developments of X-ray computed tomography over half a century: user's influence on protocol optimization. *Eur. J. Radiol.* 131: 109261. https://doi.org/10.1016/j.ejrad.2020.109261.

20 Si-Mohamed, S.A., Miailhes, J., Rodesch, P.-A. et al. (2021). Spectral photon-counting CT technology in chest imaging. *J. Clin. Med.* 10 (24): 5757. https://doi.org/10.3390/jcm10245757.

2
Conventional Computed Tomography
Essential Physics and Technology

Chapter at a Glance

Rad Tech's Guide to Photon Counting Computed Tomography,
First Edition. Euclid Seeram.
© 2025 John Wiley & Sons, Inc. Published 2025 by John Wiley & Sons, Inc.

Introduction

The use of CT imaging has increased in an exponential manner since the 1980s owing to the numerous technical advances leading to better image quality and dose optimization techniques. In the foreword of a CT textbook by Seeram [1], Dr. Patrick Brennan, Dr. Stewart Bushong, and Dr. Rob Davidson have stressed that optimizing the technology's potential requires highly efficient and knowledgeable operators. Through the years a number of significant technical advances have become available. For example, CT scanning has evolved from single-slice data acquisition to multislice data acquisition during a single breath-hold. Current state-of-the-art CT systems are based on volume data acquisition, in which the X-ray tube and detectors rotate continuously around the patient to gather transmission data from a volume of tissue rather than from one slice at a time. Furthermore, several efforts have focused on how to reduce patient dose and operate within the as low as reasonably achievable (ALARA) radiation protection principle. As a result, a number of innovative tools such as automatic exposure control (tube current modulation), automatic voltage selection (X-ray spectra optimization), more effective X-ray beam collimation, more efficient X-ray detectors, and, more recently, image reconstruction techniques based on iterative reconstruction and artificial intelligence–based reconstruction algorithms.

The purpose of this chapter is to review the essential physics of radiation attenuation in CT, followed by a brief review of the physical principles of MSCT imaging, including a review of CT image quality, in an effort to set the stage for understanding the current state-of-the-art CT technology, photon-counting CT, the details of which will be described in Chapter 3.

Radiation Attenuation Considerations in Computed Tomography: Essential Physics

Radiation attenuation is an important physics concept in CT. *Attenuation* is the reduction of the intensity of a beam of radiation as it passes through an object as illustrated in Figure 2.1, where attenuation is illustrated for two types of radiation beams (homogeneous and heterogeneous). During the development of the CT scanner, Hounsfield used a homogeneous beam from a gamma radiation source, not an X-ray tube, in his initial experiments because such a beam satisfies the requirements of the *Beer-Lambert law*. The attenuation of a homogeneous beam is exponential and follows Beer-Lambert law, expressed algebraically as:

$$I = I_0 e^{-\mu x}$$

where I is the transmitted intensity, I_0 is the original intensity, x is the thickness of the object, e is Euler's constant (2.718), and μ is the linear (per centimetre) attenuation coefficient. The objective of CT is to calculate the linear attenuation coefficients (μs) for the various tissues in the patient's anatomy. By taking the natural logarithm, μ can be solved as follows:

$$\mu = \left(I / x\right)\left(I_0 / I\right)$$

In CT, the values of I and I_0 are known since they are measured by the detectors.

Problems arising from the use of a homogeneous beam (such as, for example, the low radiation intensity) were solved using a heterogeneous beam from a diagnostic X-ray tube.

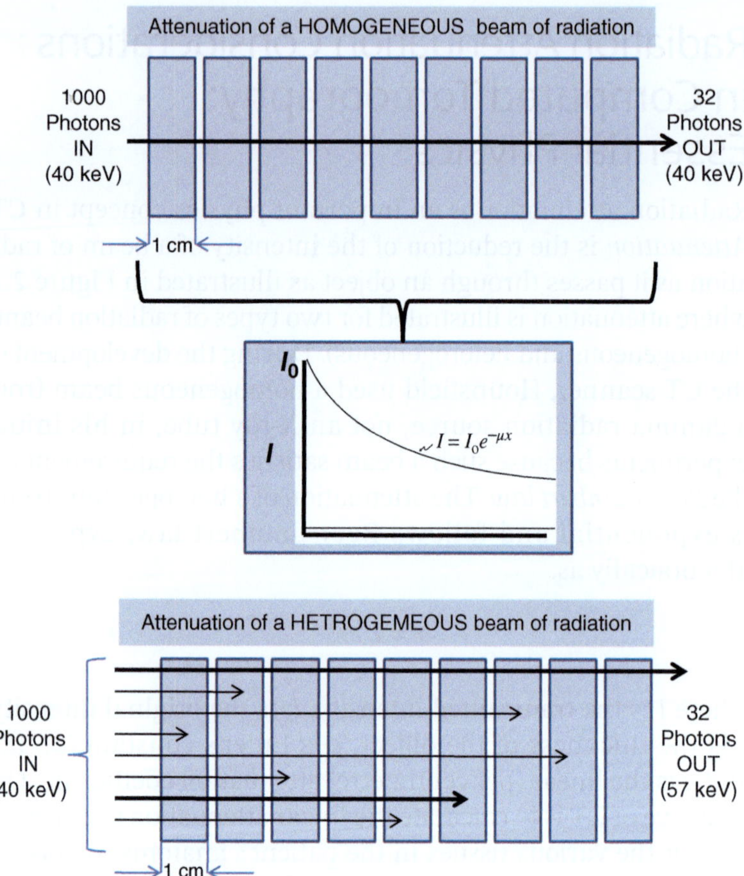

Figure 2.1 Radiation attenuation differences between a homogeneous beam and a heterogeneous beam. (See text for further explanation.)

As seen in Figure 2.1, the attenuation for a heterogeneous beam is different from that of the homogeneous beam. Equal thicknesses of material do not remove equal amounts of photons. This phenomenon results in a decrease in the number of photons (attenuation) through the object, but an increase in the energy of the attenuated photons. The latter is referred to as beam hardening and can create beam-hardening artifacts on CT images.

It is important to note that a heterogeneous beam does not satisfy the Beer-Lambert law. Therefore, Hounsfield had to make several assumptions and adjustments to determine the linear attenuation coefficients in order to satisfy the equation and solve for linear attenuation coefficient. For example, specially designed X-ray tube filters are used in CT to "trick" the detectors that a homogeneous beam is being used, thus satisfying Beer-Lambert law, and solving for attenuation coefficients of the various tissues. For a more thorough description, the interested reader should refer to Wolbarst et al. [2], Bushberg et al. [3], and Seeram [4].

Attenuation and Computed Tomography Numbers

Figure 2.2 illustrates how the attenuation values are converted into integers (0, a positive number, a negative number) referred to as CT numbers [2–4]. The system subsequently normalizes all tissue voxel values to the attenuation of water (μ_{water}). CT numbers are computed using the following relationship:

$$CT\,Number = \frac{\mu_{tissue} - \mu_{water}}{\mu_{water}} \cdot K$$

where K is the manufacturer scaling factor (contrast factor). In general, K is equal to 1000. CT numbers are also referred to as Hounsfield units (HU) to honor Hounsfield. As mentioned earlier CT numbers are always computed with reference to the attenuation of water. The CT number for water is 0, while it is +1000 for bone and −1000 for air on the Hounsfield scale.

The CT scanner obtains a matrix of CT numbers for each image slice and can be printed out as a numerical image (Figure 2.2). However, since radiologists prefer to view the gray-scale images

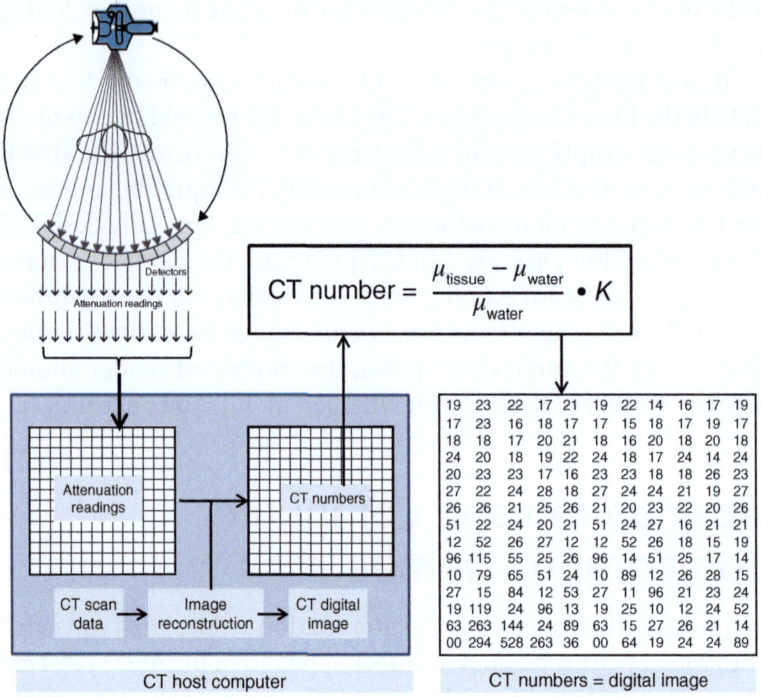

Figure 2.2 The conversion of attenuation values into integers (0, a positive number, a negative number) referred to as computed tomography (CT) numbers. The CT scanner obtains a matrix of CT numbers for each image slice and can be printed out as a numerical image.

for interpretation, the numerical image must be converted into a gray-scale image as shown in Figure 2.3. CT numbers or Hounsfield units are referred to as gray levels in digital image processing. Converting the numbers into shades of gray (gray scale) is such that the higher numbers are assigned white, lower numbers black, and gray shades between black and white. This assignment is related to the attenuation characteristics of tissues. Bone attenuates more radiation and therefore is assigned white (the bone's appearance is the same on a film-screen image as it is on a digital image).

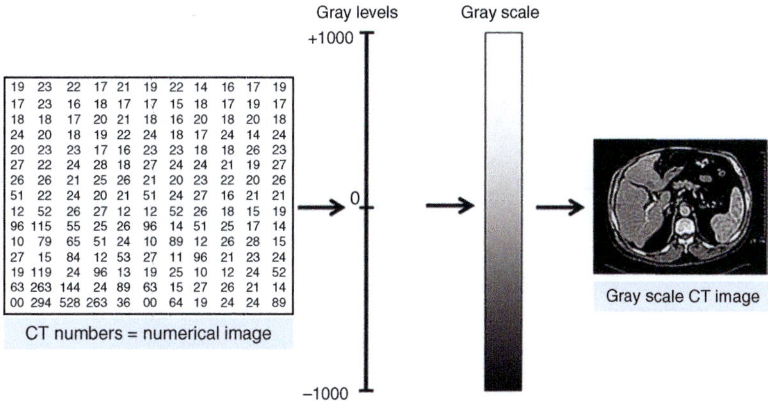

Figure 2.3 The conversion of the numerical image (computed tomography numbers) into a gray-scale image.

Air attenuates very little radiation and appears black on film-screen and digital images. The range of CT numbers is defined as the *window width*, and the center of the range is defined as the *window level*. Finally, the observer can manipulate the window width to alter image contrast, and the window level to alter image brightness.

Multislice Computed Tomography: Principles and Technology

Current CT scanners are all based on MSCT principles, for faster data acquisition, compared with earlier CT scanners. One such strategy is illustrated in Figure 2.4, which shows that the X-ray tube and detectors rotate continuously while the patient moves through the gantry. The result is increased volume coverage speed and the selection of arbitrary locations within the scanned volume of tissue during image processing. The path traced by the scanning process is called a *spiral* or *helical* path. MSCT scanners require several technical elements for successful

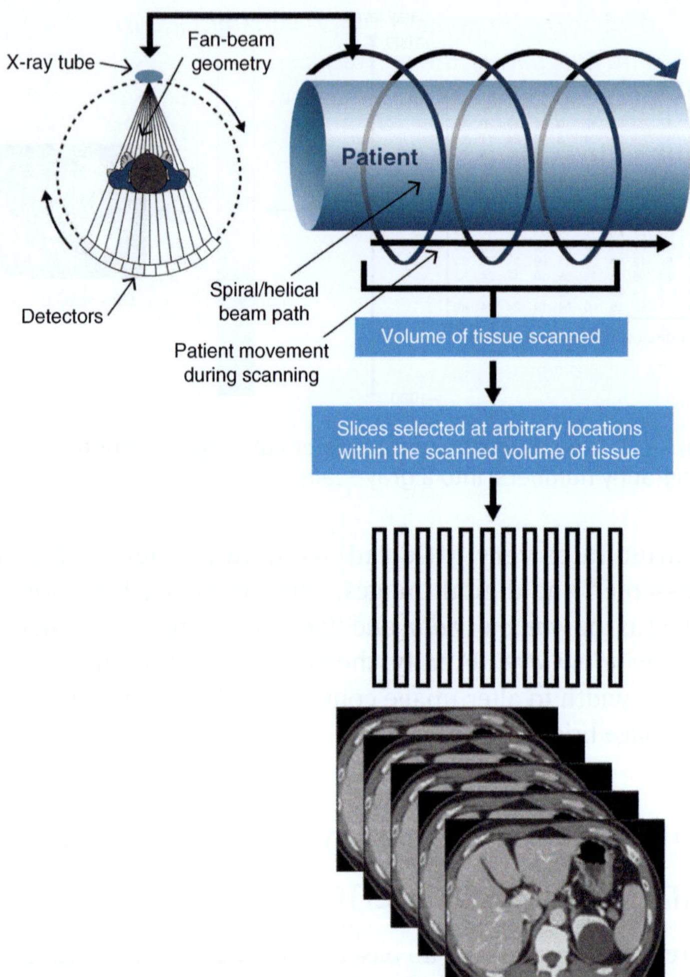

Figure 2.4 Multislice computed tomography scanners use fan-beam geometry to scan the volume of tissue.

Source: Reproduced from Seeram [5]/American Society of Radiologic Technologists.

scanning. Examples of these elements include the use of slip-ring technology, X-ray tubes that provide very high X-ray output, interpolation and image reconstruction algorithms, 2-D detector arrays, continuous table movement, and mass computer memory buffer. Of these, only the first five elements will be reviewed briefly in this chapter. Furthermore, Shefer et al. [6] in their paper on state-of-the-art CT detectors and sources states that "the three CT components with the greatest impact on image quality are the X-ray source, detection system and reconstruction algorithms." [6] For this reason, it is important to review each of these components.

Slip-Ring Technology

The slip-ring is a major system component in MSCT scanners. By definition, *slip rings* are "electromechanical devices that transmit electrical energy across a rotating interface through circular electrical conductive rings and brushes." [7] This technology allows the X-ray tube and detectors to not only rotate continuously around the patient during scanning, but also transfer the detector signals to the computer for image reconstruction.

X-Ray Tubes for Multislice Computed Tomography Scanners

X-ray tubes used in MSCT scanners feature a number of technological advances to provide higher power output and address the problems of heat generation, storage, and dissipation. For example, Fox [8] and Holmberg and Koppel [9], have identified the redesign of not only the tube envelope, cathode assembly, and anode assembly, but also the tube target. For more detailed information on MSCT X-ray tubes, the interested reader should refer to Seeram [4]. In summary, however, Seeram [4] states that "new tubes such as the Straton x-ray tube and more recently, the Vectron x-ray tube, both developed by Siemens Healthineers. These tubes are compact and use direct anode cooling technology, which results in high cooling rates and other technical advantages. Philips Healthcare has introduced the upgraded Maximus Rotalix Ceramic (iMRC) x-ray tube based on metal/ceramic technology. The iMRC also has a noiseless, spiral-groove bearing with a large liquid metal contact and a 200-mm graphite-backed, dual-suspended hydrodynamic bearing with a segmented all-metal anode disk to facilitate high heat-loading capacity and rapid heat dissipation. The upgraded tube features dynamic focal spot control, which increases the data sampling and generates ultrahigh spatial resolution while minimizing artifacts" [6].

Interpolation: An Essential Concept for Multislice Computed Tomography Imaging

In MSCT imaging, the patient moves through the gantry during the scanning process. In this respect, not all rays pass through the image plane (planar section). In non-MSCT imaging (conventional CT imaging), the reconstruction algorithm requires that data be collected from one slice, the planar section (consistent data). Therefore, in MSCT imaging, interpolation of a planar section is first required before image reconstruction. *Interpolation* is a mathematical technique for estimating the value of a function from known values on either side of it [10].

Figure 2.5 illustrates the general idea of interpolation used in MSCT imaging. A significant difference between conventional slice-by-slice CT scanning (a) and spiral/helical CT scanning (b) lies in the geometry of the slice. In (b) there is no defined slice, which results in inconsistent projection data. When inconsistent data are used with the filtered back projection (FBP) algorithm, the image displays streak artifacts similar to motion artifacts. In MSCT imaging, interpolation first produces a planar section followed by image reconstruction. The results are CT images free of motion artifacts [4].

Image Reconstruction Algorithms in a Nutshell

An *algorithm* is a finite set of rules for solving a problem. *Image reconstruction* is the heart of the CT scanner [11] and is defined as the "process of producing an image in a two-dimensional

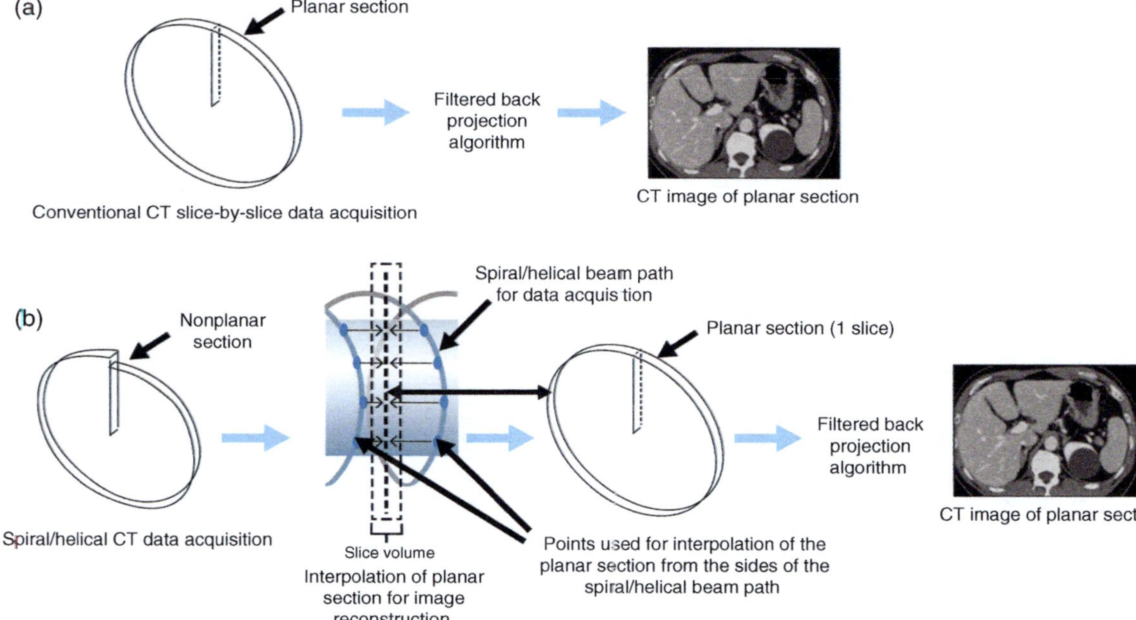

Figure 2.5 The main difference between conventional sl ce-by-slice computed tomography (CT) scanning (a) and spiral/helical CT scanning (b) lies in the geometry of the slice.

Source: Seeram [5]/American Society of Radiologic Technologists.

distribution (usually of some physical property), from estimates of its line integrals along a finite number of lines of known locations" [12]. The physical property in CT imaging is the linear attenuation coefficient (μ) of the tissues; the line integrals refer to the sum of the attenuation along each ray in the beam that passes through the slice, and the finite number of lines refer to the data collected at known positions of the X-ray tube and detectors as they rotate around the patient [11].

Through the years, there have been a number of image reconstruction algorithms used in clinical practice. Clinically useful algorithms have evolved from the FBP algorithm (which was referred to as the workhorse algorithm for several decades) and iterative reconstruction (IR) algorithms, to current state-of-the-art algorithms based on AI. By definition, an *iteration* is a calculation process using a series of operations repeated several times, until the desired output is achieved. The evolution occurred in an effort to reduce the dose to the patient through the introduction of low-dose CT (LDCT) imaging. A major problem with lowering the dose is poor image quality (noisy images). Therefore, several algorithms were developed to solve this problem when imaging at low doses, as illustrated in Figure 2.6. Low-dose imaging using the FBP algorithm results in pronounced image noise. Using IR algorithms and AI-based algorithms produced good and excellent image quality, respectively [13].

The fundamental principles of the FBP, IR, and AI-based algorithms have been described in detail by Seeram [4]. In summary, the major steps involved in the FBP algorithm and a typical IR algorithm (without modeling) are illustrated in Figure 2.7. An important difference is that while the FBP algorithm uses digital filters to produce sharp images, the IR algorithm uses accurate modeling of the CT system. For a more comprehensive description of system modeling, the interested reader may refer to Seeram [4]. All CT scanners today use IR algorithms.

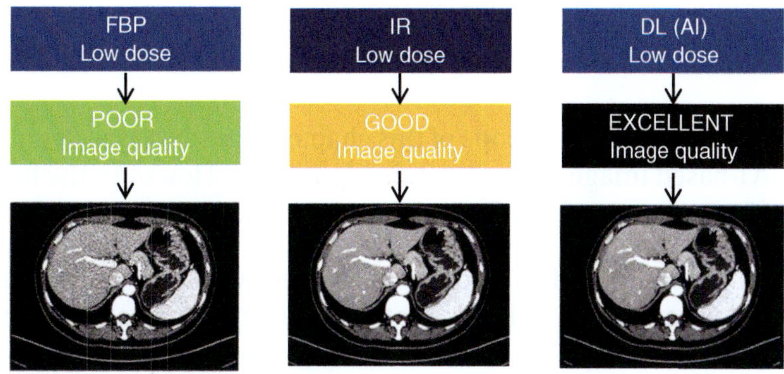

Figure 2.6 Computed tomography imaging at low dose using the filtered back projection algorithm results in pronounced image noise. The use of iterative reconstruction algorithms and artificial intelligence–based algorithms produced good and excellent image quality, respectively.

Source: Adapted from Wang et al. [13].

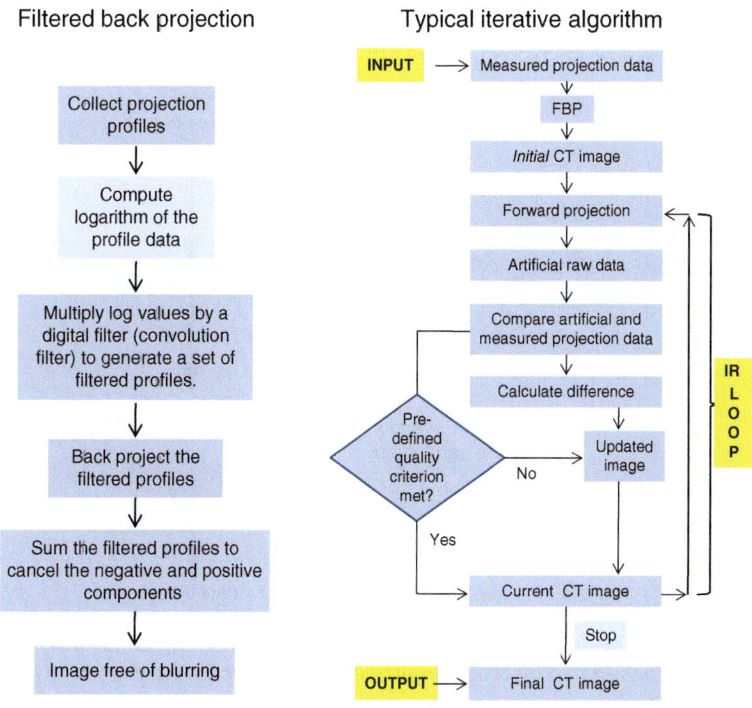

Figure 2.7 The major steps involved in the filtered back projection algorithm and a typical iterative reconstruction algorithm (without modeling). (See text for further explanation.)

It is not within the scope of this chapter to describe the details of AI-based image reconstruction algorithms. However, the following points are in order:

1. AI is a "field of science concerned with building computers and machines that can reason, learn, and act in such a way that would normally require human intelligence or that involves data whose scale exceeds what humans can analyze" [14]. Two major subfields of AI are machine learning (ML) and deep learning (DL) [11].
2. AI-based image reconstruction has been introduced in CT image reconstruction following the shortcomings of FBP and IR algorithms [11] and is graphically illustrated in Figure 2.8.

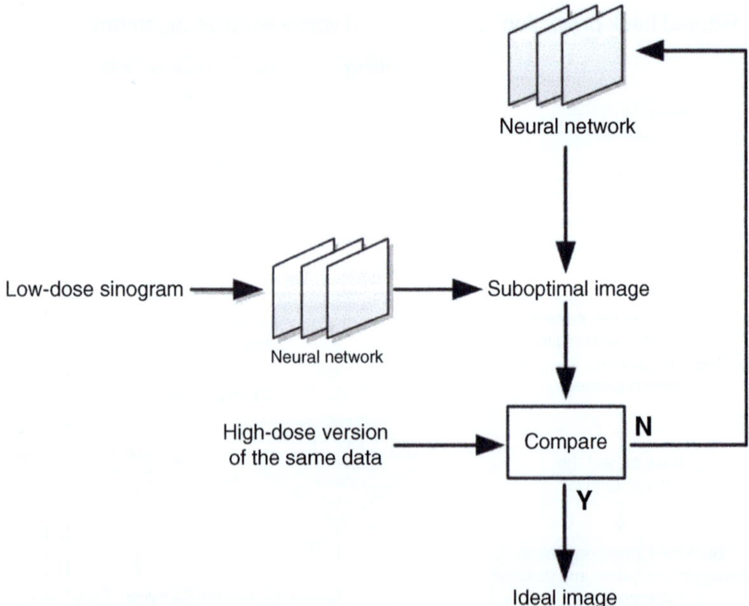

Figure 2.8 The fundamental steps involved in an artificial neural network–based reconstruction process. (See text for further explanation.)

Source: Yan et al. [17]/Tech Science Press/CC BY 4.0.

3. An AI-based reconstruction algorithm used in CT is one based on DL. This DL image reconstruction algorithm provides improved image quality as well as improved dose performance and reconstruction speed compared with iterative reconstruction methods [11]. Furthermore, DL reconstruction algorithms, when used in LDCT imaging, are intended to recognize noise from true signal and suppress the noise so anatomical and patho-logical features are clearly demonstrated, such that images show high signal-to-noise ratio.

4. In 2019, the U.S. Food and Drug Administration (U.S. FDA) approved two CT systems, namely, Advanced Intelligent Clear-IQ Engine (AiCE) [15] from Canon's Medical Systems and TrueFidelity from General Electric (GE) Healthcare [16].

5. A generalized framework for these two systems is summa-rized by Seeram [11] as follows: DR algorithm development, training and optimization of the algorithm, and verification and validation of the algorithm. The training and optimi-zation phase of the algorithm is significant. For example, while the TrueFidelity algorithm uses low- and high-dose CT data with the FBP algorithm, the AiCE algorithm uses low- and high-dose CT data with iterative reconstruction. These data sets are fed into the DL reconstruction engine (based on an artificial neural network), which produces output images with high signal-to-noise ratio.

6. The training process involves comparing output images with a reference image using various parameters, including "image noise, noise texture, low contrast resolution, and low contrast detectability. Differences are reported by the output image to the network via a technique referred to as back-propagation [11], which strengthens some equations and weakens others and tries again" This process repeats until the output image is an accurate representation of the ground truth image. Figure 2.8 summarises the basic steps involved in an artificial neural network–based reconstruction

process [17]. The network must compare its output image with a gold standard reference image (high-dose image) referred to as the *ground truth* image in order to gauge its performance (obtaining a certain level of accuracy) and learn [11].

7. During the final step, the algorithm is required to reconstruct clinical and phantom images it has never encountered, including rare cases [11].

8. More details of these DL image reconstruction algorithms, including artificial neural networks, can be found in a textbook titled *Artificial Intelligence in Medical Imaging Technology* by Seeram and Kanade [18].

Detector Technology: Key Features

Shefer et al. [6] identifies the CT detection system as one of the three components that is significant to the CT imaging process. CT detectors are coupled to the X-ray tube, capture the X-ray photons transmitted through the patient, and subsequently convert them into electrical signals. These signals are digitized and sent to the computer for image reconstruction.

There are two categories of detectors used in CT, namely, energy-integrating detectors (EIDs) and, more recently, photon-counting detectors (PCDs). EIDs are popular detectors and are used in almost all current CT scanners. While EIDs have been referred to as *indirect conversion detectors* based on the use of scintillation phosphors, PCDs are referred to as *direct conversion detectors* based on the use of semiconductors. The system components of both types of detectors are illustrated in Figure 2.9. The following points are noteworthy:

1. Scintillation crystals used in EIDs include cadmium tungstate ($CdWO_4$); ceramic material made of high-purity, rare-earth oxides based on doped rare-earth compounds such as yttria; and gadolinium oxysulfide ultrafast ceramic. The kind of scintillators used depends on the CT manufacturer.

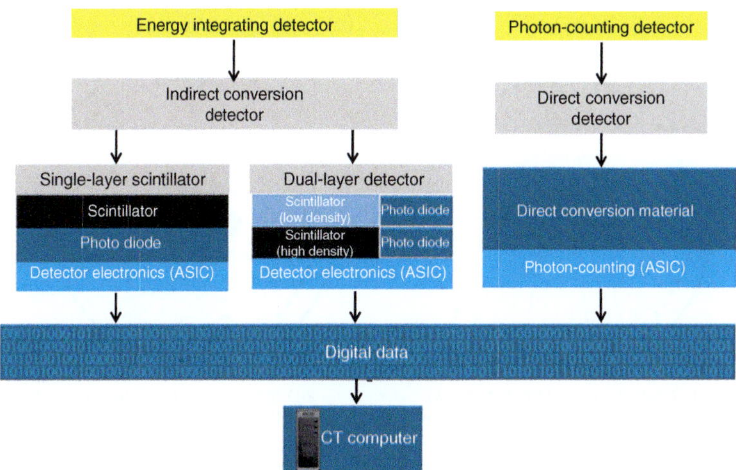

Figure 2.9 The main components of two types of detectors used in computed tomography. While energy integrating detectors are referred to as indirect conversion detectors, photon-counting detectors are referred to as direct conversion detectors. (See text for further explanation.)

For example, Philips Healthcare uses zinc selenide activated with tellurium in their dual-layer scintillator detectors [6].

2. Semiconductors such as cadmium telluride (CdTe) and cadmium zinc telluride (CZT), for example, are used in PCDs [18] because they can convert X-ray photons directly into electron hole pairs (electric charge) [19, 20].

3. The detector electronics called *application-specific integrated circuits* (ASICs) are responsible for digitizing the analog signals from the detectors.

4. MSCT scanners use 2-dimensional (2D) detector array design compared with single-slice detectors, which use 1D-detector array design, as shown in Figure 2.10. Whereas 1D detector arrays acquire 1 slice per rotation of the X-ray tube and detectors, 2D detector arrays acquire several slices per rotation of the X-ray tube and detector during scanning. For example, a 2D detector with 64 detector rows acquires 64 slices per rotation.

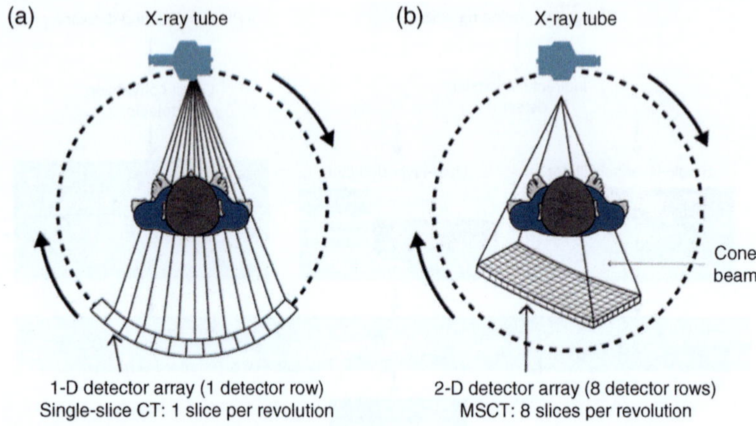

Figure 2.10 The main difference between single-slice computed tomography and multislice computed tomography (MSCT) is the detector design. Single-slice detectors are based on a 1-D detector array design (a), and MSCT detectors are based on a 2-D design (b).

Source: Seeram [5]/American Society of Radiologic Technologists.

The technical considerations of both types of CT detectors will be described further in Chapter 3.

Limitations of Energy Integrating Detectors: Image Quality Considerations

Image quality in CT is an extensive subject matter and will not be described in this book in any detail. For further details, the interested reader should refer to Wolbarst [2], Bushnerg et al. [3], and Seeram [4]. The limitations of EIDs used in conventional CT imaging have been described in the literature [19] and summarized by Flohr et al. [20] as follows: poor spatial resolution, image noise at LDCT imaging, and problems with dual-energy CT (DECT) scanning. These problems have been resolved by PCDs, which will be described in Chapter 3.

References

1 Seeram, E. (2016). *Computed Tomography: Physical Principles, Clinical Applications, and Quality Control*. Philadelphia, PA: Saunders Elsevier.

2 Wolbarst, A.B., Capasso, P., and Wyant, A.R. (2013). Computed tomography: superior contrast in three-dimensional x-ray attenuation maps. In: *Medical Imaging: Essentials for Physicians* (ed. A.B. Wolbarst, P. Capasso, and A.R. Wyant), 191–233. Hoboken, NJ: Wiley-Blackwell.

3 Bushberg, J.T., Seibert, J.A., Leidholdt, E.M., and Boone, J.M. (2012). Computed tomography. In: *The Essential Physics of Medical Imaging*, 3e, 312–374. Philadelphia, PA: Lippincott Williams & Wilkins.

4 Seeram, E. (2023). *Computed Tomography: Physical Principles, Patient Care, Clinical Applications, and Quality Control*. Philadelphia, PA: Elsevier.

5 Seeram, E. (2018). Computed tomography: a technical review. *Radiol. Technol.* 89 (3): 279–302.

6 Shefer, E., Altman, A., Behling, R. et al. (2013). State of the art of CT detectors and sources: a literature review. *Curr. Radiol. Rep.* 1 (1): 76–91. https://doi.org/10.1007/s40134-012-0006-4.

7 Brunett, C.J. (1990). *CT Design Considerations and Specifications*. Clevland, OH: Picker International.

8 Fox, S.H. (1995). CT tube technology. In: *Medical CT and Ultrasound: Current Technology and Applications* (ed. L.W. Goldman and J.B. Fowlkes), 349–357. College Park, MD: American Association of Physicists in Medicine.

9 Homberg, R. and Koppel, R. (1997). An x-ray tube assembly with rotating-anode spiral groove bearing of the second generation. *Electromedica* 66: 65–66.

10 Awati, R. (2024). What is extrapolation and interpolation? https://www.techtarget.com/whatis/definition/extrapolation-and-interpolation#. (accessed 23 September 2024).

11 Seeram, E. (2020). Computed tomography image reconstruction. *Radiol. Technol.* 92 (2): 1–15.

12 Herman, G.T. (1980). *Fundamentals of Computerized Tomography: Image Reconstruction from Projections*. New York: Academic Press.

13 Wang, S., Cao, G., Wang, Y. et al. (2021). Review and prospect: artificial intelligence in advanced medical imaging. *Front. Radiol.* 1: 781868. https://doi.org/10.3389/fradi.2021.781868.

14 What is Artificial Intelligence (AI)? https://cloud.google.com/learn/what-is-artificial-intelligence (accessed 25 September 2024).

15 Boedeker, K. (2019). AiCE deep learning reconstruction: bringing the power of ultra-high resolution CT to routine imaging. *Canon Med. Syst.* 2: 28–33.

16 Hsieh, J., Liu, E., Nett, B. et al. (2019). A new era of image reconstruction: TrueFidelity. https://www.gehealthcare.ru/-/jssmedia/040dd213fa89463287155151fdb01922.pdf (accessed 26 September 2024).

17 Yan, Q., Ye, Y., Xia, J. et al. (2023). Artificial intelligence-based image reconstruction for computed tomography: a survey. *Intell. Automat. Soft Comput.* 36 (3): 2545–2558. https://doi.org/10.32604/iasc.2023.029857.

18 Seeram, E. and Kanade, V. (2024). *Artificial Intelligence in Medical Imaging Technology: An Introduction*. Switzerland: Springer.

19 Nakamura, Y., Higaki, T., Kondo, S. et al. (2023). An introduction to photon-counting detector CT (PCD CT) for radiologists. *Jpn. J. Radiol.* 41 (3): 266–282. https://doi.org/10.1007/s11604-022-01350-6.

20 Flohr, T., Petersilka, M., Henning, A. et al. (2020). Photon-counting CT review. *Phys. Med.* 79: 126–136. https://doi.org/10.1016/j.ejmp.2020.10.030.

3 Photon-Counting Computed Tomography
Physical Principles and Technology

<table>
<tr><td colspan="2">Chapter at a Glance</td></tr>
</table>

Sections of the article titled "Photon Counting Computed Tomography" by Euclid Seeram (Directed Reading Supplement, Winter 2024) have been reprinted with permission from American Society of Radiologic Technologists. ©2020. All rights reserved.

Introduction

In Chapter 1, the invention of the CT scanner and subsequent Nobel Prize shared between CT pioneers Sir Godfrey Hounsfield and Allan Cormack were reviewed briefly. Furthermore, Chapter 1 introduced the evolution of CT detectors leading to the development of photon-counting detectors, the current state-of-the-art CT imaging technology. Chapter 2, on the other hand, provided a short review of the essential physics and technology of MSCT. Additionally, key features of CT detector technology, notably, EIDs (indirect conversion detectors), and the image quality provided by such detectors were described.

Recently, several technological developments have now enabled state-of-the-art solid-state direct conversion PCDs [1, 2]. An overview of these technical advances in CT is shown in Figure 3.1 [3]. It is important to note that currently two photon-counting CT (PCCT) scanners have been approved by the U.S. FDA for clinical use [4, 5].

The purpose of this chapter is to describe the fundamental physical principles of PCCT, including the technical design

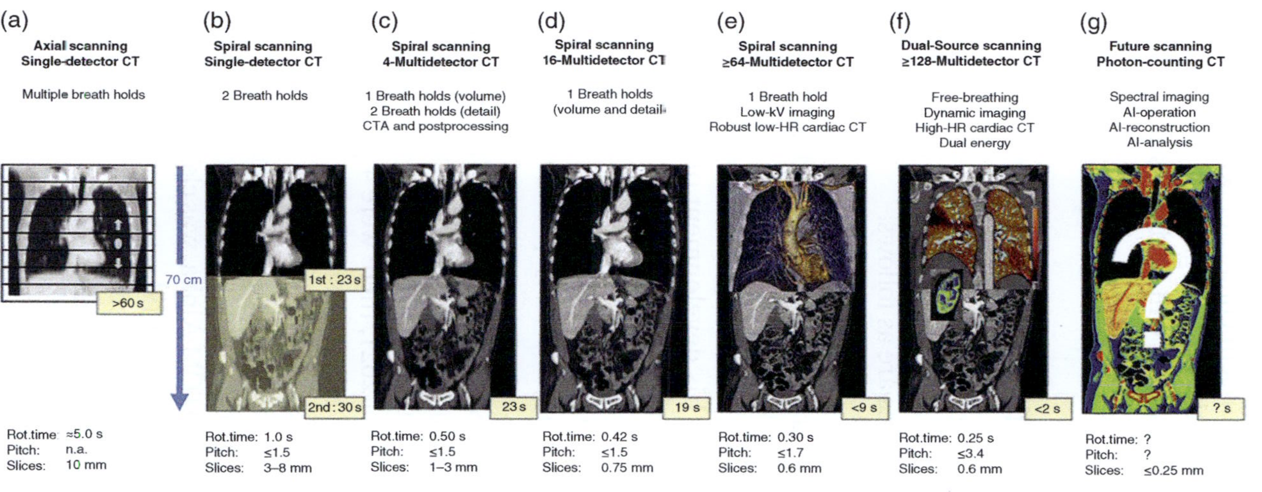

Figure 3.1 Graphical representation of the evolution of third-generation computed tomography scanner technology from a single detector row design to expected future technology (a–g).

Source: Booij et al. [3]/Elsevier/CC BY 4.0.

characteristics of their semiconductor sensors and associated electronics. Finally, the advantages of PCDs, compared with EIDs, will be listed, which will be discussed comprehensively in Chapter 4.

Historical Perspectives

The history of photon counting devices has been discussed in the literature [6, 7], and summarized briefly by Seeram [8]. A few historic features are as follows:

- The first PCDs were gas-ionization detectors, such as the Geiger–Müller counter [4].
- In 1992, Georges Charpak received the Nobel Prize in Physics for his development of the multiwire proportional chamber particle detector [6]. Later, photon counting was used in nuclear medicine with gamma cameras, also called scintillation cameras or Anger cameras, as part of early positron-emission tomography systems.
- In 2011, the U.S. FDA approved the first photon-counting imaging system, the Sectra MicroDose Mammography. Subsequently, a PCD CT imaging system using CZT was evaluated. As of 2021, there were 4 photon-counting CT systems under clinical assessment, including a mobile unit. While one system used silicon-based detectors, the others used cadmium-based detectors.
- The first photon-counting CT scanner for clinical use, the Siemens NAEOTOM Alpha, was cleared by the U.S. FDA on September 30, 2021 [9].
- The second photon-counting CT scanner became available for clinical use when NeuroLogica Corp, a subsidiary of Samsung Electronics Co. Ltd., announced its latest configuration of the mobile CT OmniTom Elite

with PCD technology, which received U.S. FDA 510(k) clearance on March 10, 2022 [5].

The interested reader should refer to Danielsson et al. [6] for further details on the history of PCDs.

Photon-Counting Detectors for Computed Tomography Imaging – Early Preclinical Works

A brief account of the application of PCDs to CT is provided by Flohr and Schmidt [10]. In summary, they noted that:

- In 2008, GE Healthcare developed the first preclinical PCD-CT prototype based on the use of a 32-row CdTe PCD.
- In 2014, Siemens Healthcare (now Siemens Healthineers) introduced three preclinical dual-source PCD-CT prototypes for clinical research purposes, using CdTe PCD.
- In 2017, Philips Healthcare employed a CZT single-source PCD-CT imaging system for research purposes using animal and human subjects.
- In 2020, Siemens Healthcare (now Siemens Healthineers) installed second-generation single-source PCD-CT scanners, in three clinical facilities "used to evaluate the performance and image quality of PCD-CT in a general clinical setting" [10].
- Finally, in 2021, Siemens Healthineers introduced the first commercial first-generation PCD dual-source CT (PCD-DSCT) with two CdTe detectors. This scanner is called NAEOTOME Alpha, approved by the U.S. FDA on September 30, 2021, for clinical use (as mentioned earlier).

The interested reader should refer to the article by Flohr and Schmidt [10] and Ballabriga et al. [11] for further details on various physical parameters such as gantry rotation, collimation, pixel characteristics, field-of-view (FOV), and z-coverage.

Computed Tomography Detectors: Physical Principles and Technology

Currently, there are two types of detectors used in CT, based on how X-ray photons are converted into electrical signals [11]. These include indirect conversion detectors and direct conversion detectors. While the former is also referred to as EIDs, the latter is known as PCDs, as schematically outlined in Figure 3.2. Both detectors convert X-ray photons to electrical signals. However, EIDs use scintillators to first convert X-ray photons to light,

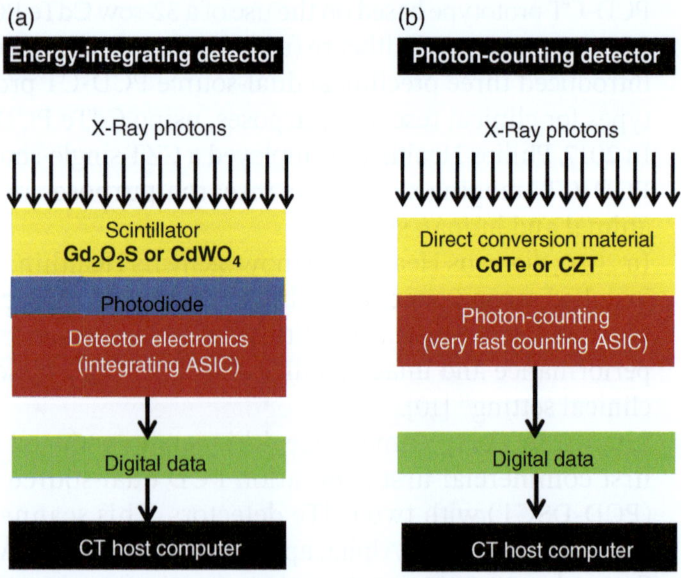

Figure 3.2 A schematic overview of two types of detectors used in computed tomography, based on how X-ray photons are converted into electrical signals: the indirect conversion detectors (a) and direct conversion detectors (b). See text for further explanation.

then the photodiode converts the light into electrical signals (Figure 3.2a). This light conversion process is missing in the PCD, which converts X-ray photons directly into electrical signals using semiconductors (Figure 3.2b).

A notable distinction between the EID and the PCD is schematically shown in Figure 3.3. While Figure 3.3a (EID) shows that all measured photons in one projection are *integrated* to create the pulse signals of that projection, Figure 3.3b illustrates that the measured photons are separated out into individual pulse signals. This principle leads to several advantages of PCDs over EIDs.

Energy-Integrating Detectors

Conventional CT scanners use EIDs, including DSCT scanners [1, 2, 12, 13]. As illustrated in Figure 3.4, there are three major system components, namely, the solid-state scintillator, a photodiode, and the processing electrical circuit. The detector works as follows:

1. The solid-state scintillator (gadolinium oxysulfide or cadmium tungstate [12]; others such as lutetium-based or yttrium-based garnet, gadolinium oxysulfide ceramic, and praseodymium gadolinium oxysulfide ceramic [14]) converts X-ray photons into light photons. The number of light photons emitted is directly proportional to the energy of the X-ray photons falling on the scintillator.
2. Light photons fall upon the photodiode, which converts them into electrical signals.
3. These electrical signals are sent to the processing circuit.
4. The components of the processing circuit include an amplifier, a signal-integrating ASIC, and an analog-to-digital converter (ADC). The ADC samples the electrical signal from the integrator circuit and converts it into digital data, which are subsequently processed using the image reconstruction algorithm.

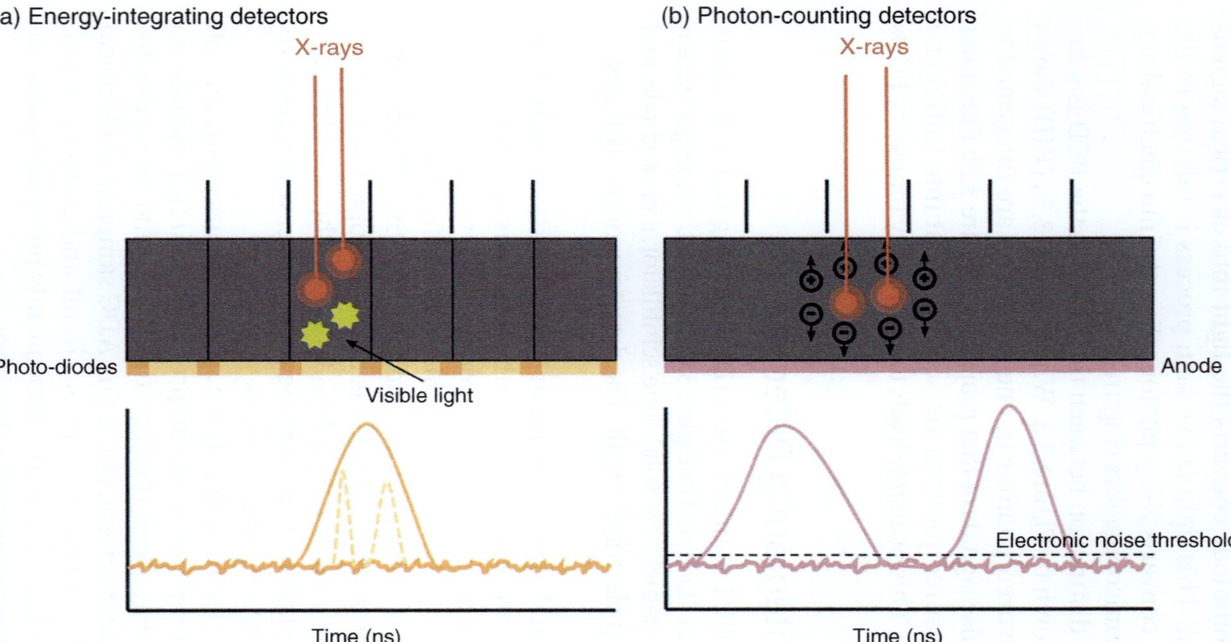

Figure 3.3 A notable distinction between the energy-integrating detectors (EIDs) and the photon-counting detector (PCD). While (a) (EID) shows that all measured photons in one projection are integrated to create the pulse signals of that projection, (b) illustrates that the measured photons are separated out into individual pulse signals. This principle leads to several advantages of PCDs over EIDs.

Source: van der Bie et al. [26]/Elsevier/CC BY 4.0.

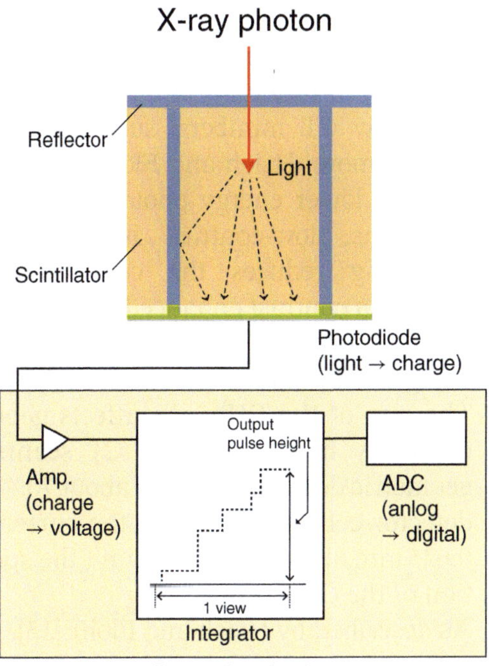

Figure 3.4 The basic structural components of an energy-integrating detector. Reprinted under the creative commons 4.0 international license.

Source: Nakamura et al. [12]/Springer Nature/CC BY 4.0.

5. There are three important points to consider when using EIDs:

   A. The beam from the X-ray tube is heterogeneous (consists of high-energy and low-energy photons), and because the light emitted from the scintillator is directly proportional to the energy of the photons, that is high-energy photons produce more light than low-energy photons, high-energy photons produce more electronic signals. This creates an imbalance known as the *energy-weighting* situation. Low-energy photons create low electronic signals (which are easily distorted by electronic noise) increasing overall image noise at lower x-ray doses and reducing image quality of tissues with low CT numbers, such as the lungs [13]. Furthermore, Hsieh and Flohr [15] point out that because lower energy photons carry most of the soft-tissue, low-contrast information, "energy-weighting reduces the contrast-to-noise ratio mainly in contrast enhanced CT scans because the x-ray absorption of iodine is highest at lower energies (above its K-edge at 33 keV)" [15].

B. The size of the EID cells affects geometric dose efficiency in CT. Modern CT scanners have a geometric dose efficiency of about 70% to 80%, and detector cells smaller than the current size (0.5–0.625 mm at the isocenter) limit the spatial resolution of the CT scanner [13].

C. As described by Hsieh and Flohr [15].

The individual detector cells are separated by optically opaque reflection layers based on TiO_2 (Titanium Dioxide) or Cr_2O_3 (Chromium Oxide) to prevent optical crosstalk (Figure 3.5). They have a width of about 0.1 mm and reduce the geometric dose efficiency of the detector. X-ray photons absorbed in the separation layers do not contribute to the measured signal even though they have passed through the patient. Current medical CT detectors with an active cell size of about $0.8 \times 0.8 – 1 \times 1\ mm^2$ have a geometric dose efficiency of 70%–80%. If the width of the separation layers is kept constant, significantly reducing the size of the cells (in order to increase the spatial resolution) would further decrease the geometric efficiency – therefore, it is challenging to increase the spatial resolution of solid-state scintillation detectors.

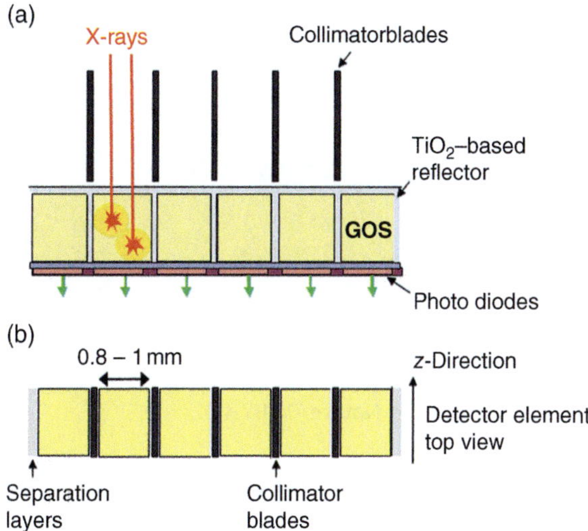

Figure 3.5 Schematic drawing of an energy-integrating scintillator detector: (a) side view and (b) top view. The z direction is the patient's longitudinal direction. Detector cells made of a scintillator such as GOS absorb the X-rays (red arrows) and convert their energy into visible light (orange circles).

Source: Hsieh and Flohr [15]/SPIE/CC BY 4.0.

The limitations of EIDs have been discussed in the literature [1, 2, 6, 10, 12, 13]. For example, Flohr et al. [13] summarize these shortcomings as limited spatial resolution, image noise at low X-ray doses, and problems with DSCT imaging. Figure 3.6 illustrates the limited spatial resolution and image noise between an EID and a PCD.

Photon-Counting Detectors

PCDs are referred to as direct conversion detectors because they convert X-ray photons directly into electrical signals. PCDs are designed not only to count single photons from the X-ray beam, but also to measure their energies individually. PCDs overcome many of the shortcomings of EIDs and offer several advantages

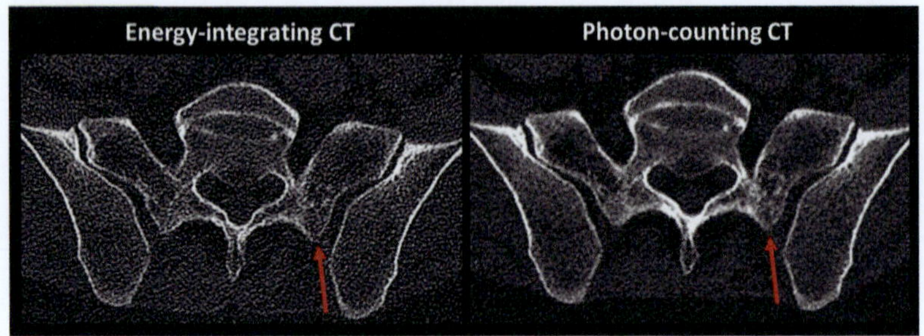

Figure 3.6 The limited spatial resolution and image noise between an energy-integrating detector and a photon-counting detector.
Source: Rau et al. [27]/Springer Nature/CC BY 4.0.

compared with EIDs [1, 2, 6, 10, 12, 13, 15]. These will be listed later in the chapter.

Photon-Counting Detectors: Physical Principles and Technology

An important characteristic of PCDs is that they must be able to count single photons from the X-ray beam very quickly and measure their energy individually. Many of the limitations of EIDs are overcome by PCDs owing to the nature of the physics and technological design of their semiconductor sensors and associated electronics. Photon-counting CT "is a promising technology that might substantially improve and expand the applicability of CT imaging" [16].

The following subsection will describe the essential structural and functional elements of PCDs.

Basic Structure and Function of a Photon-Counting Detector

The fundamental structure of a PCD is shown in Figure 3.7. There are two major system components, namely, the semiconductor (sensor) and the electrical processing circuit.

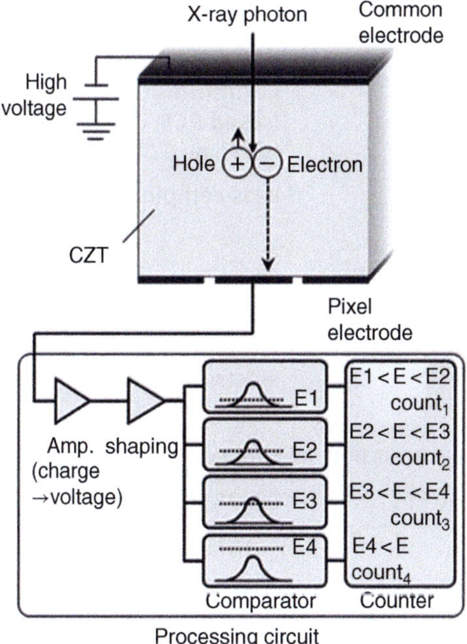

Figure 3.7 The basic structural components of a photon-ounting detector. *Source:* Nakamura et al. [12]/Springer Nature/CC BY 4.0.

Semiconductors for PCDs are selected on the basis of several physical characteristics such as high X-ray absorption efficiency and high atomic number [6, 10, 12]. Presently, two semiconductor materials are used in PCCT scanners, namely, cadmium (zinc) telluride (CdTe or CZT) and silicon (Si). Greffier et al. [17] provides a comparison of characteristics between cadmium-based and silicon-based detectors outlined in Table 3.1. Furthermore, Greffier et al. [17] identifies and describes the main characteristics of current prototype, preclinical or clinical PCCT systems suitable for clinical imaging, from Siemens Healthineers, Samsung Healthcare, MARS Bioimaging Limited, Canon Medical Systems, Philips Healthcare, and GE Healthcare.

Table 3.1 Comparison of characteristics between cadmium-based and silicon-based detectors.

Characteristic	Cadmium-based PCD (CdTe or CZT)	Silicon-based PCD
Manufacturing complexity	Less complex	More complex
Thickness (orientation)	Face-on (1.4–2 mm)	Edge-on (30–60 mm)
Photo-electric effect/ compton effect	Photo-electric effect predominant	Compton effect predominant
k-Fluorescence emission	Higher	Lower
Lowest energy bin	20–25 keV	5–10 keV
Energy resolution (FWHM)	5–10 keV	3–5 keV
Spatial resolution	Higher	Lower
Energy-resolving capabilities	Lower	Higher

CdTe, cadmium telluride; CZT, cadmium zinc telluride; FWHM, full width at half maximum; PCD, photon-counting detector.
Source: Greffier et al. [17]/Elsevier/CC BY 4.0.

Exposure of the Semiconductor

When X-ray photons fall upon the semiconductor, a physical interaction occurs, which creates *electron–hole pairs* [18]. The physical interaction is such that an electron (negatively charged subatomic particle) in the valence band acquires enough energy to jump into the conduction band, thus leaving a hole in the valence band, thus creating an electron–hole pair [19]. This is a fundamental role in the electrical properties of semiconductors. These electron–hole pairs create an electron charge cloud that is proportional to the energy of the photon striking the semiconductor, and this negatively charged cloud is attracted to the positively charged anode of the detector, called a pixel electrode. Additionally, "the electrons drift to the anodes and induce short-current pulses in the order of nanoseconds (ns). A pulse-shaping circuit transforms them to voltage pulses" [15]. Charge clouds produce electrical signals or pulses. One charge cloud produces one pulse, as shown in Figure 3.8. Although hundreds of millions of these interactions occur per square millimeter per second, the PCD can register each pulse [12].

Figure 3.9 shows a side view (a) and a top view (b) of a direct converting PCD. An important point to consider is that the electron–hole pairs are separated in a strong electric field between cathode and pixelated anodes. A potential subpixel structure is indicated for the three left detector cells. The pixelated anodes must then be correspondingly structured (not shown in the figure). Smaller pixel sizes can be obtained with PCDs because

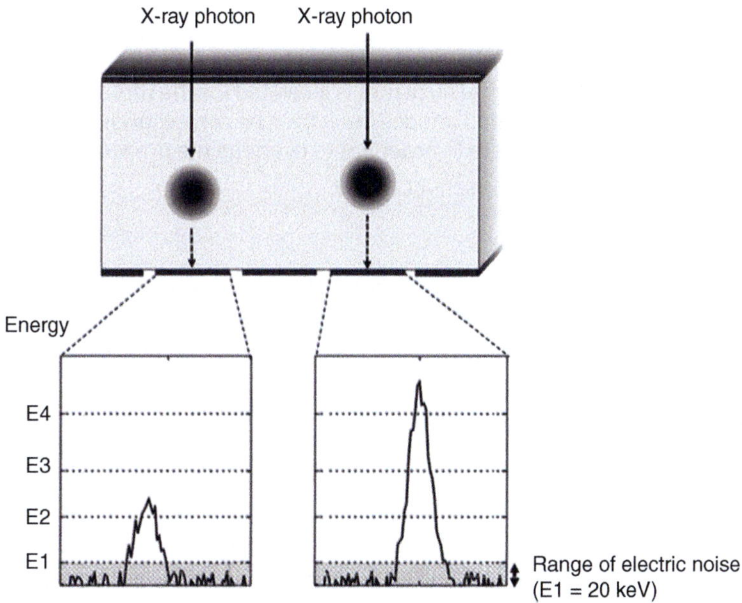

Figure 3.8 X-ray photons falling on the semiconductor detector produce electron–hole pairs (charge cloud).

Source: Nakamura et al. [12]/Springer Nature/CC BY 4.0.

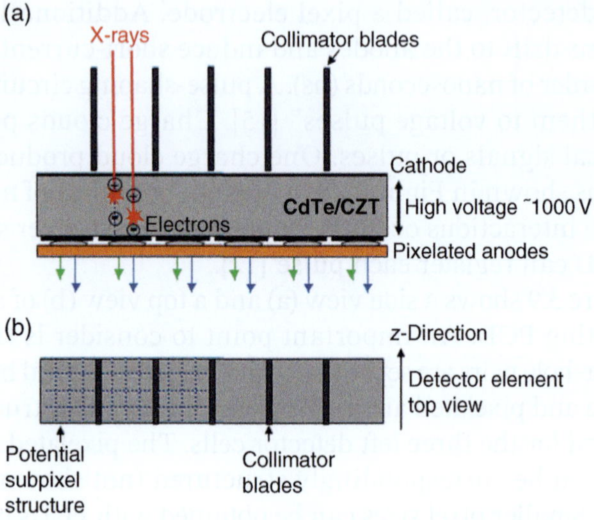

Figure 3.9 Schematic drawing of a direct converting photon-counting detector: (a) side view and (b) top view. The X-rays (red arrows) absorbed in a semiconductor such as CdTe or CZT produce electron–hole pairs that are separated in a strong electric field between cathode and pixelated anodes. A potential subpixel structure is indicated for the three left detector cells. The pixelated anodes must then be correspondingly structured (not shown here in order not to overload the drawing).

Source: Hsieh and Flohr [15]/SPIE/CC BY 4.0.

there are no gaps or separators between detector elements, as is the case with EIDs (Figure 3.4). Smaller pixel sizes produce better spatial resolution.

Electrical Processing Circuit

The next system component is the electrical processing circuit. Unlike EIDs, which requires an integrating ASIC, PCDs require a very fast counting ASIC. As shown in Figure 3.7, the circuit is coupled to the semiconductor pixel electrode and consists of amplifiers, comparator circuits, and counters. As described by Hsieh et al. [19] a PDC detector is made up of hundreds of thousands of pixels and each pixel is coupled to an individual processing electrical circuit (Figure 3.7). It is not within the scope of this book to describe the details of the electrical processing circuit. However, the following points are noteworthy:

1. The intensity of pulses (electrical signals) is compared by the comparator circuit to a reference voltage referred to as the *energy threshold.*
2. When detected pulses exceed this energy threshold, the comparator circuit activates and increments its counter [6, 19].
3. As shown in Figure 3.7, each pixel has four comparator circuits set to different energy thresholds (E_1, E_2, E_3, and E_4) and four counters that track the results from the comparators. Each comparator/counter pair tracks the number of pulses above a certain wave height, proportional to the absorbed photon energy. Because each counter tracks a different wave height, the approximate energy level of each photon is also noted, allowing multiple energy discrimination. In other words, PCDs count individual photons and allocate them to predetermined energy thresholds and bins as shown in Figure 3.10.

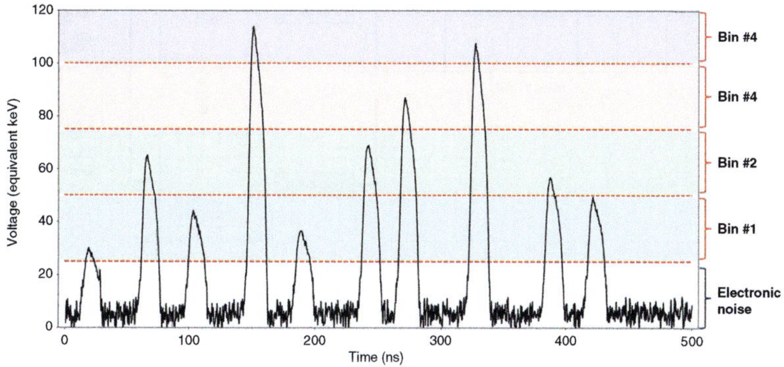

Figure 3.10 Example of a 500-ns signal output of a photon-counting detector pixel.

Source: Si-Mohamed et al. [21]/MDPI/CC BY 4.0.

Additionally, "the photon-counting design allows the generation of *energy-selective images*, from which a set of material concentration maps can be obtained. Material concentration maps can then be combined in different ways to obtain monochromatic images, virtual non-contrast images, or material-specific color-overlay images," [20] as illustrated in Figure 3.11.

4. The design of the comparators ensure that PCDs inherently have excellent noise reduction, in low-dose

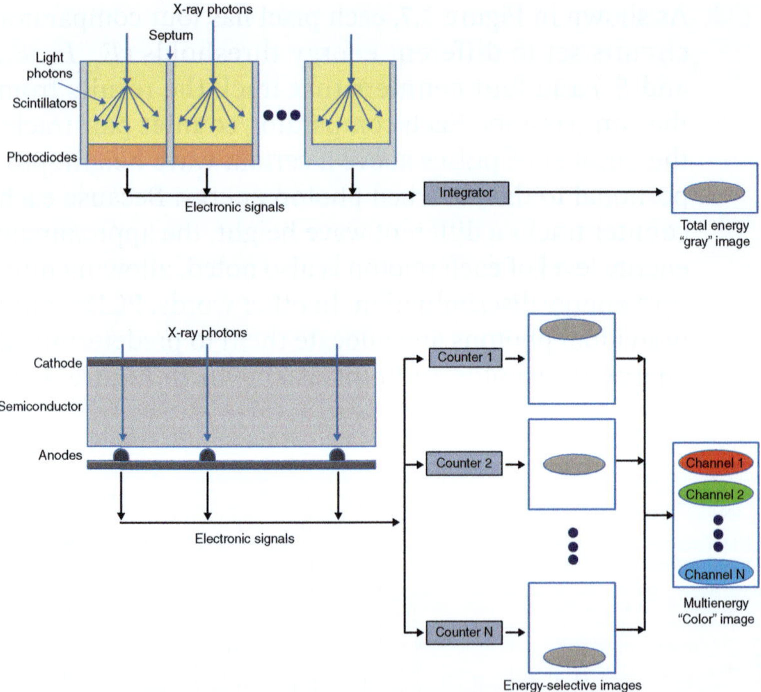

Figure 3.11 Schematic representation of an energy-integrating detector (top) and of a photon-counting detector directly converting X-rays into an electrical signal (bottom). The photon-counting design allows the generation of energy-selective images, from which a set of material concentration maps can be obtained. Material concentration maps can then be combined in different ways to obtain monochromatic images, virtual noncontrast images, or material-specific color-overlay images.

Source: Meloni et al. [20]/MDPI/CC BY 4.0.

CT imaging. Furthermore, less streak artifacts and more stable CT numbers result when scanning obese patients [15]. Electronic noise (from the hardware electronics) is present when the photon energy is less than 20 keV, so electronic noise can be filtered out entirely by tuning the lowest energy threshold of the comparators to about 20 keV [6, 17, 19, 21].

Image Reconstruction in Photon-Counting Computed Tomography

As described in Chapter 2, image reconstruction in CT using EIDs involves the use of several reconstruction algorithms such as the FBP algorithm, IR algorithms, and AI-based image reconstruction methods. In PCCT systems, new image reconstruction algorithms have been introduced to handle the increased complexity of the data set, the acquisition of spectral information, and the noise model used in PCCT systems [22–24]. One such algorithm is the *quantum iterative reconstruction* (QIR), which is complex and not within the scope of this book. However, the following is noteworthy: QIR uses an iterative reconstruction method for statistical optimization of spectral data and corrects for geometric artifacts [22].

The QIR algorithm features four levels of strength (QIR-1, QIR-2, QIR-3, and QIR-4) that can be applied to the reconstructed images with respect to noise reduction. The visual effect of each of these QIR levels on a CT image is shown in Figure 3.12.

Advantages of Photon-Counting Computed Tomography at a Glance

PCDs offer several advantages compared with EIDs. These advantages have been described in the literature and include dose reduction, low-dose imaging, electronic noise removal, improved spatial resolution, weighting of photons, improved

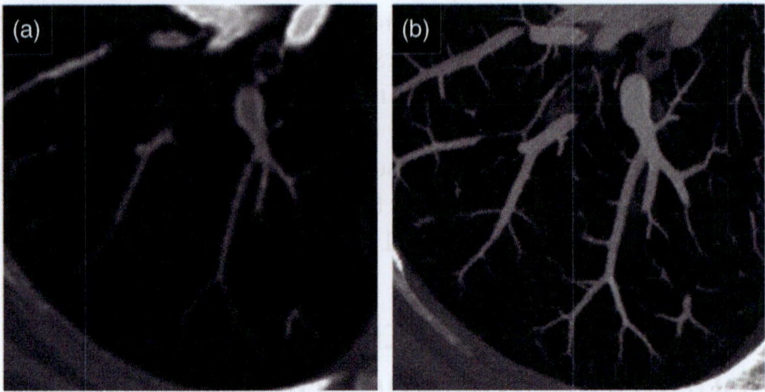

Figure 3.12 Comparison of the distal arterial pulmonary tree imaged with a dual-layer energy-integrating detector computed tomography (a) and a clinical prototype photon-counting detector computed tomography (b), after injection of iodinated contrast agent. The improvement in quality is visible, notably of the distal vessel lumen and calipers that are depicted until the pleural space.

Source: Si-Mohamed et al. [21]/MDPI/CC BY 4.0.

contrast resolution, and material-specific imaging [12–17, 19]. For example, improved spatial resolution of the PCD is shown in Figure 3.13 showing a comparison of the distal arterial pulmonary tree imaged with a dual-layer EID-CT scanner (a) and a clinical prototype PCD-CT scanner (b). These advantages will be discussed and illustrated in more detail in Chapter 4.

Technical Limitations of Photon-Counting Detectors

The technical limitations of PCDs for use in CT imaging have been identified in the literature as early as 2013 by Taguchi and Iwanczyk [25], in an article titled "Vision 20/20: Single Photon Counting X-Ray Detectors in Medical Imaging" published in *Medical Physics*. Later, more articles identified and described these limitations [6, 12, 13, 15–17]. A summary of several of these is illustrated in Figure 3.14, including pile-up, charge sharing, k-escape, and Compton scattering effects.

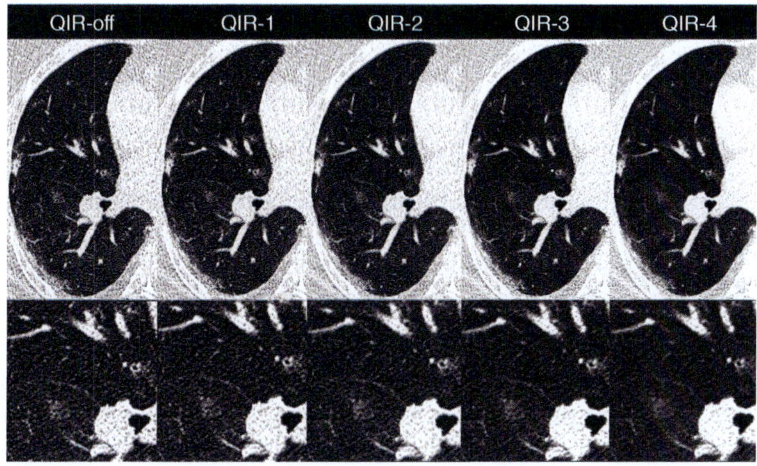

Figure 3.13 Images of a 55-year-old female patient with atypical pneumonia. Noise was reduced considerably when changing from QIR-off to higher levels of QIR, that is QIR-1, QIR-2, QIR-3, and QIR-4. *Source:* Sartoretti et al. [23]/MDPI/CC BY 4.0.

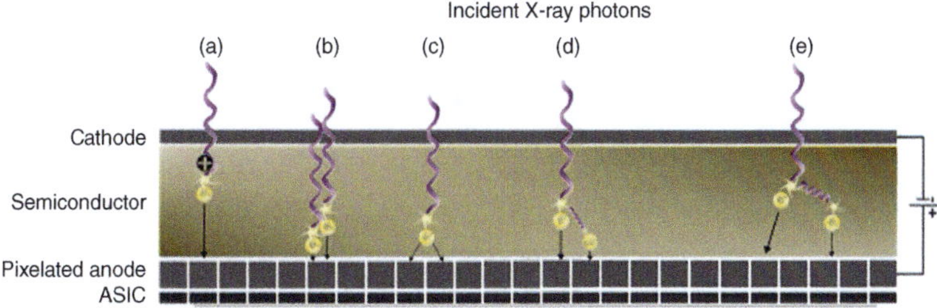

Figure 3.14 A summary of pile-up, charge sharing, k-escape, and Compton scattering effects. *Source:* Greffier et al. [17]/Elsevier/CC BY 4.0.

The following explanations of each of these effects is quoted directly from Greffier et al. [17]:

- *Pulse Pile-Up*: The pile-up effect occurs when "multiple x-ray photons arrive at the detector within a short time, causing overlapping signals and compromising accurate energy measurement" [17].

- *Charge Sharing*: Charge sharing effect arises "when the charge generated by a single X-ray photon is distributed between two detector elements, leading to reduced spatial and energy resolution" [17].
- *K-escape*: K-escape effect occurs "when a new charge cloud is generated by the Kα X-ray fluorescence of the sensor materials (CdTe or Si) and registered by a pixel as two separate events" [17].
- *Compton Scattering*: Compton scattering effects occur "when any secondary photons produced in the semi-conductor material is registered by the same pixel or an adjacent pixel as two separate events, yielding to a lower record of the real energy value" [17].

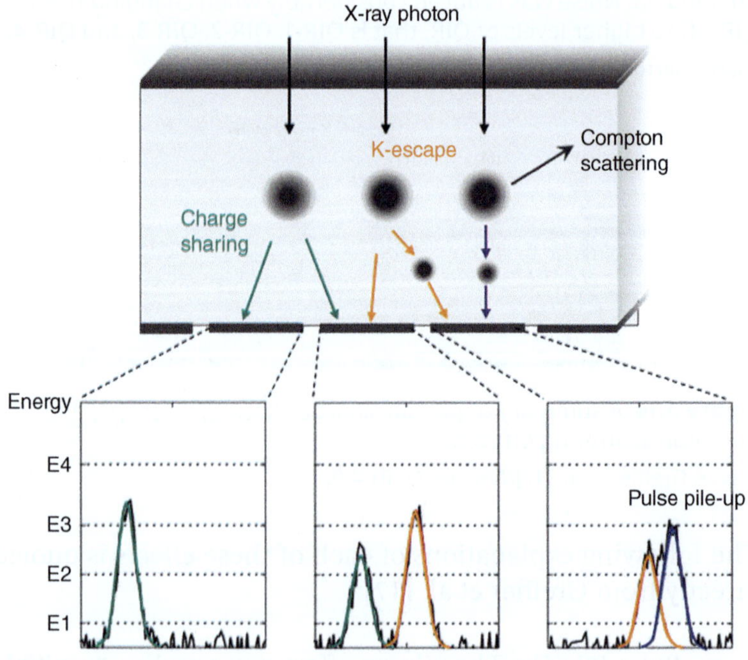

Figure 3.15 Charge sharing, K-escape, and Compton scattering cause inaccurate signal measurements in the photon-counting detector.

Source: Nakamura et al. [12]/Springer Nature/CC BY 4.0.

The physical processes of charge-sharing, K-escape, and Compton scattering will result in what is referred to as *crosstalk*, which leads to inaccurate signal acquisition, as schematically shown in Figure 3.15. Crosstalk occurs when a single photon interacts with more than one pixel, resulting in more than one count or an inaccurate energy evaluation [12, 15].

References

1 Willemink, M.J., Persson, M., Pourmorteza, A. et al. (2018). Photon-counting CT: technical principles and clinical prospects. *Radiology* 289 (2): 293–312. https://doi.org/10.1148/radiol.2018172656.

2 Leng, S., Bruesewitz, M., Tao, S. et al. (2019). Photon-counting detector CT: system design and clinical applications of an emerging technology. *Radiographics* 39 (3): 729–743. https://doi.org/10.1148/rg.2019.180115.

3 Booij, R., Budde, R.P.J., Dijkshoorn, M.L., and van Straten, M. (2020). Technological developments of X-ray computed tomography over half a century: user's influence on protocol optimization. *Eur. J. Radiol.* 131: 109261. https://doi.org/10.1016/j.ejrad.2020.109261.

4 Siemens Healthineers announces FDA 510(k) clearance of Naeotom Alpha, the world's first photon-counting CT. https://www.siemens-healthineers.com/press/releases/naeotomfda (accessed 2 October 2024).

5 NeuroLogica Corp receives FDA 510(k) clearance for enhanced OmniTom Elite with ultra-high resolution PCD technology. https://www.neurologica.com/publications/press-releases/neurologica-receives-innovative-technology-designation-from-vizient-0 (accessed 2 October 2024).

6 Danielsson, M., Persson, M., and Sjölin, M. (2021). Photon-counting x-ray detectors for CT. *Phys. Med. Biol.* 66 (3): 03TR01. https://doi.org/10.1088/1361-6560/abc5a5.

7 Charpak, G. (1997). Electronic imaging of ionizing radiation with limited avalanches in gases. *Rev. Mod. Phys.* 65: 591. https://doi.org/10.1103/RevModPhys.65.59.

8 US Food and Drug Administration (2024). FDA clears first major imaging device advancement for computed tomography in nearly a decade. https://www.fda.gov/news-events/press-announcements/fda-clears-first-major-imaging-device-advancement-computed-tomography-nearly-decade (accessed 2 October 2024).

9 Seeram E. (2023). Photon counting computed tomography. ASRT Essential Education. CE Directed Reading (November 2023).

10 Flohr, T. and Schmidt, B. (2023). Technical Basics and Clinical Benefits of Photon-Counting CT. *Investig. Radiol.* 58 (7): 441–450.

11 Ballabriga, R., Alozy, J., Bandi, F.N. et al. (2021). Photon counting detectors for X-ray imaging with emphasis on CT. *IEEE Trans. Rad. Plasma Med. Sci.* 5 (4): 422–440, 2021. https://doi.org/10.1109/TRPMS.2020.3002949.

12 Nakamura, Y., Higaki, T., Kondo, S. et al. (2023). An introduction to photon-counting detector CT (PCD CT) for radiologists. *Jpn. J. Radiol.* 41 (3): 266–282. https://doi.org/10.1007/s11604-022-01350-6.

13 Flohr, T., Petersilka, M., Henning, A. et al. (2020). Photon-counting CT review. *Phys Med.* 79: 126–136. https://doi.org/10.1016/j.ejmp.2020.10.030.

14 Seeram, E. (2023). *Computed Tomography: Physical Principles, Patient Care, Clinical Applications, and Quality Control,* 5e. Elsevier.

15 Hsieh, J. and Flohr, T. (2021). Computed tomography recent history and future perspectives. *J Med Imaging (Bellingham)* 8 (5): 052109. https://doi.org/10.1117/1.JMI.8.5.052109.

16 Sartoretti, T., Wildberger, J.E., Flohr, T., and Alkadhi, H. (2023). Photon-counting detector CT: early clinical experience review. *Br. J. Radiol.* 96 (1147): 20220544. https://doi.org/10.1259/bjr.20220544.

17 Greffier, J., Viry, A., Robert, A. et al. (2024). Photon-counting CT systems: A technical review of current clinical possibilities. *Diagn. Interv. Imaging* https://doi.org/10.1016/j.diii.2024.09.002.

18 Luiz, H.G., Kociak, T. and M. Quantum. (2017). Nanooptics in the Electron Microscope Advances in Imaging and Electron Physics, 199: 185–235. Cambridge, MA. Academic Press is an imprint of Elsevier.

19 Hsieh, S.S., Leng, S., Rajendran, K. et al. (2021). Photon counting CT: clinical applications and future developments. *IEEE Trans. Radiat. Plasma Med. Sci.* 5 (4): 441–452. https://doi.org/10.1109/TRPMS.2020.3020212.

20 Meloni, A., Frijia, F., Panetta, D. et al. (2023). Photon-counting computed tomography (PCCT): technical background and cardio-vascular applications. *Diagnostics* 13 (4): 645. https://doi.org/10.3390/diagnostics13040645.

21 Si-Mohamed, S.A., Miailhes, J., Rodesch, P.-A. et al. (2021). Spectral photon-counting CT technology in chest imaging. *J. Clin. Med.* 10 (24): 5757. https://doi.org/10.3390/jcm10245757.

22 Woeltjen, M.M., Niehoff, J.H., Michael, A.E. et al. (2022). Low-dose high resolution photon-counting CT of the lung: radiation dose and image quality in the clinical routine. *Diagnostics (Basel)* 12 (6): 1441. https://doi.org/10.3390/diagnostics12061441.

23 Sartoretti, T., Racine, D., Mergen, V. et al. (2022). Quantum iterative reconstruction for low-dose ultra-high-resolution photon-counting detector CT of the lung. *Diagnostics (Basel)* 12 (2): 522. https://doi.org/10.3390/diagnostics12020522.

24 Shanblatt, E., O'Doherty, J., Petersilka, M. et al. (2022). NAEOTOM alpha with quantum technology. Siemens Healthcare white paper.

25 Taguchi, K. and Iwanczyk, J.S. (2013). Vision 20/20: single photon counting x-ray detectors in medical imaging. *Med. Phys.* 40 (10): 100901.

26 van der Bie, J., van Straten, M., Booij, R. et al. (2023). Photon-counting CT: review of initial clinical results. *Eur. J. Radiol.* 163: 110829.

27 Rau, A., Straehle, J., Stein, T. et al. (2023). Photon-Counting Computed Tomography (PC-CT) of the spine: impact on diagnostic confidence and radiation dose. *Eur. Radiol.* 33: 5578–5586. https://doi.org/10.1007/s00330-023-09511-5.

4 Advantages of Photon Counting Computed Tomography

Introduction

The advantages of PCCT have been described extensively in the literature [1–12]. Advantages of PCCT imaging, compared with EID-CT imaging, as identified by these papers include improved spatial resolution, electronic noise removal, improved contrast resolution via energy weighting, dose reduction, and material-specific imaging, with each advantage offering

Rad Tech's Guide to Photon Counting Computed Tomography,
First Edition. Euclid Seeram.
© 2025 John Wiley & Sons, Inc. Published 2025 by John Wiley & Sons, Inc.

unique clinical applications [2]. For example, the advantage of high spatial resolution opens possible applications in temporal bone, musculoskeletal, lung, and cardiovascular imaging, such as stent imaging, and in CT pediatric imaging [13]. High spatial resolution is of "particular interest for these anatomical areas because the clear depiction of fine details may effectively enhance diagnostic accuracy" [12]. Furthermore, the advantages of reduced electronic noise, photon weighting, and material-specific imaging are useful in imaging patients who are obese in low-dose CT imaging; in contrast-enhanced CT for abdominal, neurologic, and cardiovascular exams; and for future clinical applications in plaque and bone evaluation, virtual no-contrast and noncalcium imaging, as well as virtual monoenergetic synthesis, respectively [2].

The purpose of this chapter is to present a broad overview of the advantages of PCCT systems, compared with CT systems using EIDs and to illustrate each advantage with select anatomical areas, in an effort to enhance diagnostic interpretation of clinical images.

Advantages of Photon-Counting Detectors

Higher/Improved Spatial Resolution

As described in Chapter 3, spatial resolution is a primary factor in CT image quality and is affected by the size of the detector. In general, smaller detector sizes allow for more detector elements, better spatial resolution, and sharper images. Specifically, PCDs do not use septa to separate detector elements as is the case with EIDs, and hence the detector elements can be smaller and more densely populated [14, 15]. This means that PCD-CT imaging systems can produce images with high spatial resolution, as demonstrated in

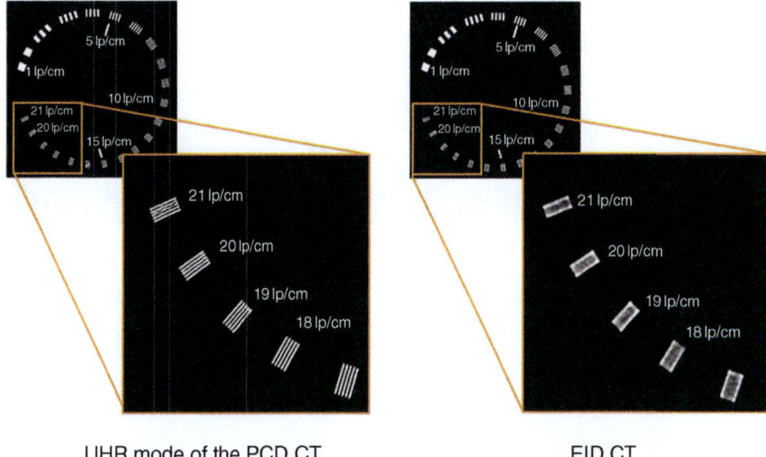

Figure 4.1 Comparison of spatial resolution in the phantom images between ultra-high-resolution (UHR) mode of the photon-counting detector computed tomography (PCD-CT) and energy-integrating detector computed tomography (EID-CT) (using author's own unpublished data) systems. The phantom used for this imaging is Catphan 500 with CTP528 High-Resolution Module (Phantom Laboratory Inc., Greenwich, USA).

Source: Nakamura et al. [5]/Springer Nature/CC BY 4.0.

Figures 4.1 and 4.2. While the former shows images of a Catphan 500 High-Resolution Module discriminating bar patterns up to 21-line pairs per centimeter (lp/cm) compared with the EID, the latter shows images of a fish demonstrating the degree of sharpness (high spatial resolution) of the PCD-CT detector element compared with the EID-CT detector element [5].

This higher spatial resolution characteristic of PCDs have been shown to be beneficial when "evaluating small structures and for identifying coronary artery calcium and coronary artery plaques, diagnosing lung lesions and temporal bone lesions" [5].

One example to illustrate this advantage is a clinical study by Woeltjen et al. [16], titled "Low-Dose High-Resolution Photon-Counting CT of the Lung: Radiation Dose and Image Quality

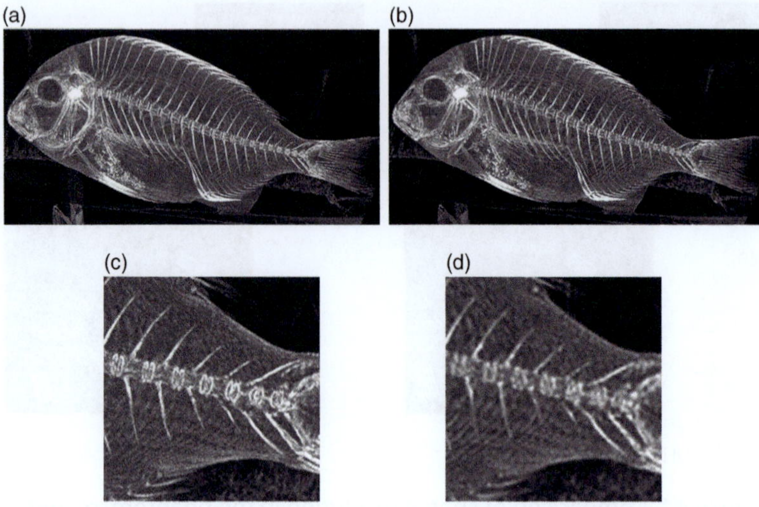

Figure 4.2 Maximum-intensity projection images of fish (using author's own unpublished data). (a) Photon-counting detector computed tomography (PCD CT) image in high-resolution mode (matrix: 1024 × 1024, slab thickness: 45.75 mm). (b) PCD CT image with low resolution equivalent to conventional energy-integrating detector computed tomography (matrix: 512 × 512, slab thickness: 45.75 mm). (c) Magnification of (a). (d) Magnification of (b). The overall structure is sharply delineated in (a) and (c) compared with (b) and (d).

Source: Nakamura et al. [5]/Springer Nature/CC BY 4.0.

in the Clinical Routine." This study, which investigated both the qualitative and quantitative image quality of low-dose high-resolution lung CT scans acquired with the first clinically approved PCCT scanner, shows the improved spatial resolution of a PCCT system compared with an EID-CT system (Figure 4.3). Another example of this advantage is a study by Hermans et al. [17], which showed that PCD-CT images of the temporal bone structures provided "better visualization" compared with current generation multidetector EID-CT images as demonstrated in Figure 4.4.

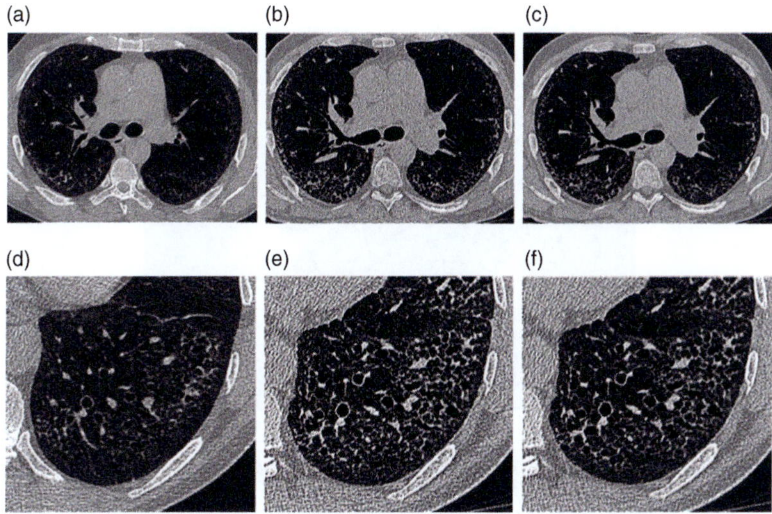

Figure 4.3 Images of the whole lung (a–c) and enlarged image sections (d–f) of the same patient. (a, d) Were created with an energy-integrating detector computed tomography (EID-CT) scanner; (b, e) were created with a photon-counting detector computed tomography (PCD-CT) scanner without an iterative reconstruction algorithm (QIR–); (c, f) are PCD-CT images reconstructed with an iterative reconstruction algorithm (QIR+).

Source: Woeltjen et al. [16]/MDPI/CC BY 4.0.

Electronic Noise Removal

A significant advantage of PCDs is reduction of electronic noise, and as such "the image quality of low-dose-scans and scans of patients with a large body size is improved" [5]. In high-dose imaging, electronic noise can be disregarded since quantum noise predominates. Electronic noise, however, "cannot be ignored when the radiation dose is low. Electronic noise is usually observed as pulses with an energy lower than 20 keV" [5]. In PCD imaging, by setting the lowest counter energy threshold to just above the level of electronic noise (about 20 keV), as shown in Figure 4.5, electronic noise can be removed. Removing such

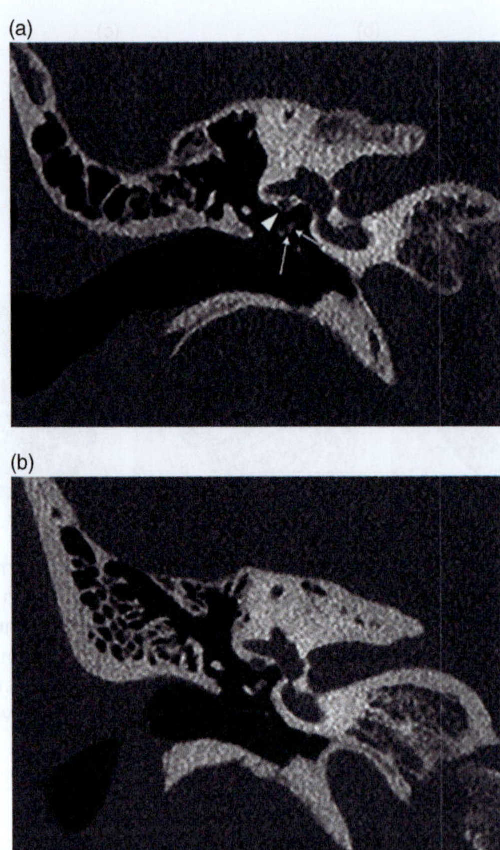

Figure 4.4 Coronal reformatted Multidetector Computed Tomography (MDCT) using energy-integrating detectors (EIDs) (a) and photon-counting computed tomography (PCCT) (b) image through right temporal bone. Incudostapedial joint (left arrow), stapedial head (right arrow), and cortical lining of tympanic segment of facial nerve canal (arrowhead) are labeled. The PCCT images were scored higher with "excellent visibility" by observers compared with the MDCT using EIDs images, which were scored as "recognizable" or "clearly recognizable."

Source: From Hermans et al. [17]/Springer Nature/CC BY 4.0.

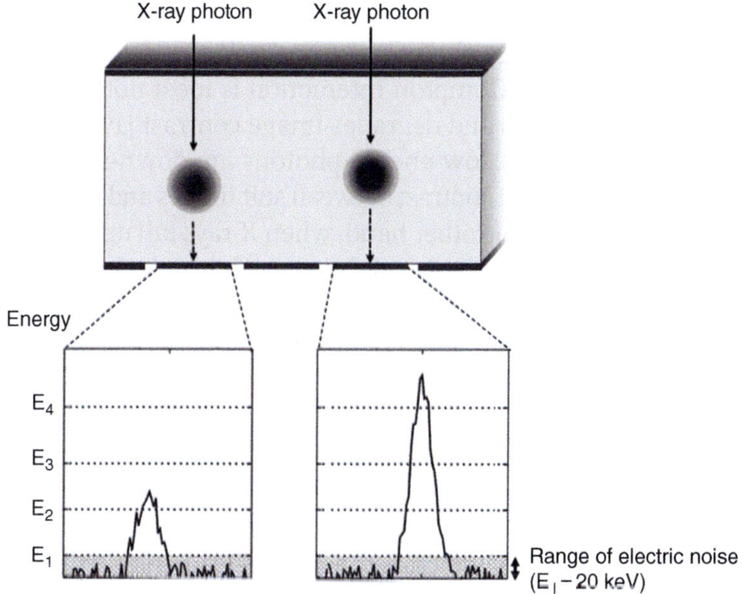

Figure 4.5 X-ray photons falling on the semiconductor detector produce electron–hole pairs (charge cloud).

Source: Nakamura et al. [5]/Springer Nature/CC BY 4.0.

noise improves the quality of CT images when the scanner is operated in low-dose imaging mode [5–7].

Energy Weighting/Improved Contrast Resolution

One of the key characteristics of PCDs is that they enable photon *energy weighting,* referred to as "a kind of reconstruction method for Spectral CT" [18], which can improve image contrast and reduce image noise by assigning different weights to different photon energies. The X-ray beam from the X-ray tube consists of low- and high-energy photons, some of which interact with patient tissues through the photoelectric absorption and

Compton scattering. While the former interaction is most notable on low-energy photons and has a pronounced effect on image contrast, the Compton interaction is most notable with high-energy photons and degrades image contrast [19, 20].

When using EIDs, low-energy photons are down-weighted, thus degrading image contrast between soft tissues and iodinated contrast media. On the other hand, when X-rays fall upon PCDs, all photons receive uniform weighting, and thus the image contrast between soft tissues and iodinated contrast is increased [7, 10, 11, 16]. Furthermore, the literature reports that the contrast-to-noise ratio (CNR) among soft tissues is also improved when low-energy photon weighting is increased [10, 11, 21]. PCD technology allows the user to define weights (in keV) before scanning to optimize the value of particular exams [2, 22].

A detailed description of energy weighting is not within the scope of this book. However, two common methods that are pixel based include projection-based energy weighting and image-based energy weighting. While the former uses the measured projection data set, the latter uses the reconstructed radiation attenuation coefficients [18]. The latter method is illustrated in Figure 4.6. The "projected images of each energy region are normalized and individually reconstructed using filtered back projection (FBP). The weighting factors are obtained from CT images of each energy bin, and the reconstructed images are weighted and summed, during which process the weighting factors are calculated by contrast and noise information provided by the images" [18].

Increased Dose Efficiency

PCCT offers increased dose efficiency, that is, the ability of the PCD to detect X-ray photons more efficiently [15] compared with EIDs. Since PCDs do not have an antiscatter grid, 100% of the photons fall upon the detector surface, resulting in this major advantage [23, 24]. Additionally, this dose efficiency is

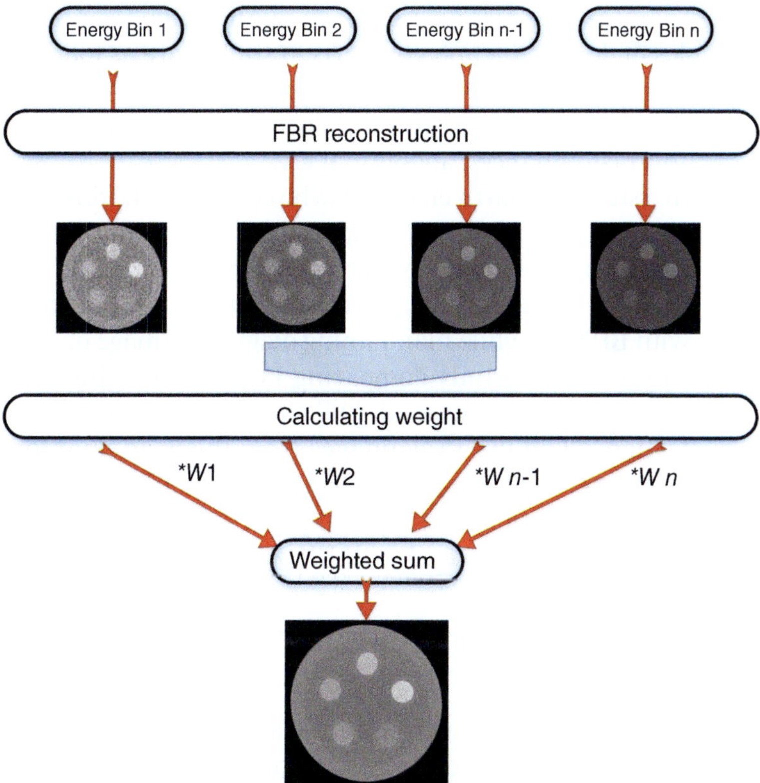

Figure 4.6 The major steps of the image-based energy weighting in photon-counting computed tomography. See text for further explanation.

Source: Reproduced from Zhiwei et al. [18]/NDT.net.

attributed to electrical noise removal, energy weighting, and no detector septa [25].

The advantage of dose reduction using PCDs has been discussed in the literature for various anatomical examinations, such as the abdomen [25], the lumbar spine [26], sinus and temporal bone imaging [27], and pediatric cardiothoracic CT imaging [28]. These studies showed significant dose reduction while maintaining diagnostic image quality. Representative examples of dose-reduction comparison studies are as follows:

1. Onishi et al. [25] showed a dose reduction of 32% for contrast-enhanced abdominal CT.
2. In a study by Marth et al. [26], who compared the dose and image quality of PCD-CT and EID-CT of the lumbar spine using tin filtration in both imaging modalities, found that PCD-CT resulted in significantly lower dose compared with EID-CT while maintaining diagnostic image quality.
3. In yet another study comparing PCD-CT imaging with EID-CT, Rajendran et al. [27] showed that with tin filtration, "The PCD-CT images from the head phantom and the cadaver scans demonstrated a dose reduction of 67% and 83%, for sinus and temporal bone examinations, respectively, compared with EID-CT" [27].

Correction of Beam-Hardening Artifacts

Artifacts common to imaging with CT systems using EIDs include beam-hardening artifacts, metal artifacts, partial volume artifacts, and ring artifacts, and they have been described in the literature [18, 28]. CT systems using PCDs, artifacts such as beam hardening, and metal implants can be reduced since high-energy pulses counted in the higher energy bins are less susceptible to beam hardening compared with the low-energy pulses [2, 5, 7, 25, 26, 29, 30]. "In particular, PCDs demonstrate optimal immunity to beam-hardening effects when employing high-energy thresholds" [30]. Additionally, ring artifacts in PCD-CT can be successfully removed [31–33].

Material-Specific Imaging/Multienergy Acquisition

One of the major imaging features of PCCT systems is that of material decomposition using specialized algorithms called

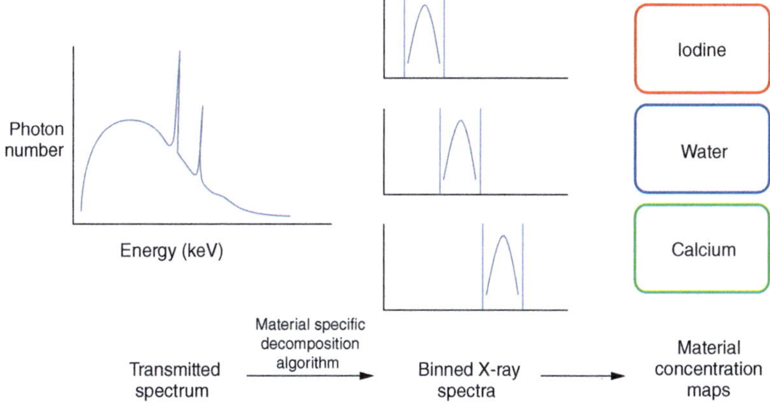

Figure 4.7 Graphical representation of material-specific imaging enabled by spectral information.
Source: Tortora et al. [22]/MDPI/CC BY 4.0.

material decomposition algorithms, which "break down unknown tissues into specific materials, based on their unique x-ray attenuation characteristics at various energy levels ... to generate *material-specific images,* which can display and measure the presence of particular elements in a CT volume, and energy-selective images" [30]. This process is illustrated in Figure 4.7.

Additionally, the multienergy acquisition feature of PCCT systems enables *K-edge imaging* [30], which is described as "the possibility of adding additional materials to the spectral decomposition of the images based on their distinct K-edge energies ... and relies on adjusting the acquisition energy thresholds to capture the target materials' unique energy shifts at the K-edge. K-edge imaging represents a 'breakthrough' in CT since it provides 'opportunities for the use of non-iodine contrast agents, such as gold, silver, platinum, bismuth, and ytterbium, and for the development of new types of contrast agents, such as nanoparticles targeted to particular cells or enzymes'" [30].

In conclusion, compared to EID-CT imaging PCD-CT imaging systems offer improved image quality (contrast and spatial resolution) at lower doses. Furthermore, PCD-CT offers not only energy weighting but also quantitative imaging and material decomposition. Clinical examinations that may benefit from these improvements include cardiovascular, neurological, thoracic, and abdominal applications, as well as pediatric and oncology exams. These applications will be highlighted in Chapter 6.

References

1 Willemink MJ, Persson M, Pourmorteza A, Pelc NJ, Fleischmann D. Photon-counting CT: technical principles and clinical prospects. *Radiology* 2018;289(2):293–312. doi:https://doi.org/10.1148/radiol.2018172656

2 Leng, S., Bruesewitz, M., Tao, S. et al. (2019). Photon-counting detector CT: system design and clinical applications of an emerging technology. *Radiographics* 39 (3): 729–743. https://doi.org/10.1148/rg.2019,180115.

3 Si-Mohamed, S.A., Miailhes, J., Rodesch, P.-A. et al. (2021). Spectral photon-counting CT technology in chest imaging. *J. Clin. Med.* 10 (24): 5757. https://doi.org/10.3390/jcm10245757.

4 McCollough, C.H., Leng, S., Yu, L., and Fletcher, J.G. (2015). Dual- and multienergy CT: principles, technical approaches, and clinical applications. *Radiology* 276 (3): 637–653. https://doi.org/10.1148/radiol.2015,142631.

5 Nakamura, Y., Higaki, T., Kondo, S. et al. (2023). An introduction to photon-counting detector CT (PCD CT) for radiologists. *Jpn. J. Radiol.* 41 (3): 266–282. https://doi.org/10.1007/s11604-022-01350-6.

6 Flohr, T., Petersilka, M., Henning, A. et al. (2020). Photon-counting CT review. *Phys. Med.* 79: 126–136. https://doi.org/10.1016/j.ejmp.2020.10.030.

7 Danielsson, M., Persson, M., and Sjölin, M. (2021). Photon-counting x-ray detectors for CT. *Phys. Med. Biol.* 66 (3): 03TR01. https://doi.org/10.1088/1361-6560/abc5a5.

8 Bartlett, D.J., Koo, C.W., Bartholmai, B.J. et al. (2019). High-resolution chest computed tomography imaging of the lungs: impact of 1024 matrix reconstruction and photon-counting detector computed tomography. *Investig. Radiol.* 54 (3): 129–137. https://doi.org/10.1097/RLI.0000000000000524.

9 Zhou W, Lane JI, Carlson ML, et al. Comparison of a photon counting-detector CT with an energy-integrating-detector CT for temporal bone imaging: a cadaveric study. *AJNR Am. J. Neuroradiol.* 2018;39(9):1733-1738. https://doi.org/10.3174/ajnr.A5768

10 Esquivel, A., Ferrero, A., Mileto, A. et al. (2022). Photon-counting detector CT: key points radiologists should know. *Korean J. Radiol.* 23 (9): 854–865. https://doi.org/10.3348/kjr.2022.0377.

11 Kalluri, K.S., Mahd, M., and Glick, S.J. (2013). Investigation of energy weighting using an energy discriminating photon counting detector for breast CT. *Med. Phys.* 40 (8): 081923. https://doi.org/10.1118/1.4813901.

12 Sartoretti, T., Wildberger, J.E., Flohr, T., and Alkadhi, H. (2023). Photon-counting detector CT: early clinical experience review. *Br. J. Radiol.* 96 (1147): 20220544. https://doi.org/10.1259/bjr.20220544.

13 Aliukonyte, L., Caudri, D., Booij, R. et al. (2024). Unlocking the potential of photon counting detector CT for paediatric imaging: a pictorial essay. *BJR|Open* 6 (1): tzae015. https://doi.org/10.1093/bjro/tzae015.

14 Baek, J., Pineda, A.R., and Pelc, N.J. (2013). To bin or not to bin? The effect of CT system limiting resolution on noise and detectability. *Phys. Med. Biol.* 58 (5): 1433–1446. https://doi.org/10.1088/0031-9155/58/5/1433.

15 Pourmorteza, A., Symons, R., Reich, D.S. et al. (2017). Photon-counting CT of the brain: in vivo human results and image-quality assessment. *AJNR Am. J. Neuroradiol.* 38 (12): 2257–2263. https://doi.org/10.3174/ajnr.A5402.

16 Woeltjen, M.M., Niehoff, J.H., Michael, A.E. et al. (2022). Low-dose high-resolution photon-counting CT of the lung: radiation dose and image quality in the clinical routine. *Diagnostics* 12: 1441. https://doi.org/10.3390/diagnostics12061441.

17 Hermans, R., Boomgaert, L., Cockmartin, L. et al. (2023). Photon-counting CT allows better visualization of temporal bone structures in comparison with current generation multi-detector CT. *Insights Imaging* 14: 112. https://doi.org/10.1186/s13244-023-01467-w.

18 Zhiwei, C., Mohan, L., Zhidu, Z. et al. (2019). Study on Energy Weighting Imaging Technology in Multispectral CT. 9th Conference on Industrial Computed Tomography (iCT) 2019,

13-15 Feb, Padova, Italy. *e-J. Nondestruct. Test.* 24 (3): https://doi.org/10.58286/23744.

19 Bushong, S. (2021). *Radiologic Science for Technologists. Physics, Biology, and Protection*, 12e. St Louis, MO: Elsevier.

20 Bushberg, J.T., Seibert, A.J., Leidholdt, E.M. Jr., and Boone, J.M. (2021). *The Essential Physics of Medical Imaging*, 4e. Philadelphia, PA: Wolters Kluwer|Lippincott Williams & Wilkins.

21 Shikhaliev, P.M. (2005). Beam hardening artefacts in computed tomography with photon counting, charge integrating and energy weighting detectors: a simulation study. *Phys. Med. Biol.* 50 (24): 5813–5827. https://doi.org/10.1088/0031-9155/50/24/004.

22 Tortora, M., Gemini, L., D'Iglio, I. et al. (2022). Spectral photon-counting computed tomography: a review on technical principles and clinical applications. *J Imaging.* 8 (4): 112. https://doi.org/10.3390/jimaging8040112.

23 Symons, R., Pourmorteza, A., Sandfort, V. et al. (2017). Feasibility of dose-reduced chest CT with photon counting detectors: initial results in humans. *Radiology* 285: 980–989.

24 Pourmorteza, A., Symons, R., Henning, A. et al. (2018). Dose efficiency of quarter millimeter photon-counting computed tomography: first-in-human results. *Investig. Radiol.* 53: 365–372.

25 Onishi, H., Tsuboyama, T., Nakamoto, A. et al. (2024). Photon-counting CT: technical features and clinical impact on abdominal imaging. *Abdom. Radiol.* 49: 4383–4399. https://doi.org/10.1007/s00261-024-04414-5.

26 Marth, A.A., Marcus, R.P., Feuerriegel, G.C. et al. (2024). Photon-counting detector CT versus energy-integrating detector ct of the lumbar spine: comparison of radiation dose and image quality. *Am. J. Roentgenol.* 222: e232995. https://doi.org/10.2214/AJR.23.29950AJR.

27 Rajendran, K., Voss, B.A., Zhou, W. et al. (2020). Dose reduction for sinus and temporal bone imaging using photon-counting detector CT with an additional tin filter. *Investig. Radiol.* 55 (2): 91–100. https://doi.org/10.1097/RLI.0000000000000614.

28 Seeram, E. (2023). Computed tomography: physical principles, patient care, clinical applications, and quality control. Maryland, MO.

29 Siegel, M.J. and Ramirez-Giraldo, J.C. (2024). Photon counting detector computed tomography in pediatric cardiothoracic CT imaging. *Radiol. Adv.* 1 (2): umae012. https://doi.org/10.1093/radadv/umae012.

30 Meloni, A., Maffei, E., Clemente, A. et al. (2024). Spectral photon-counting computed tomography: technical principles and applications in the assessment of cardiovascular diseases. *J. Clin. Med.* 13 (8): 2359. https://doi.org/10.3390/jcm13082359.

31 Schmidt, T.G., Sammut, B.A., Barber, R.F. et al. (2022). Addressing CT metal artifacts using photon-counting detectors and one-step spectral CT image reconstruction. *Med. Phys.* 49 (5): 3021–3040. https://doi.org/10.1002/mp.15621.

32 Zhou, W., Bartlett, D.J., Diehn, F.E. et al. (2019). Reduction of metal artifacts and improvement in dose efficiency using photon-counting detector computed tomography and tin filtration. *Investig. Radiol.* 54 (4): 204–211. https://doi.org/10.1097/RLT.0000000000000535.

33 An, K., Wang, J., Zhou, R. et al. (2020). Ring-artifacts removal for photon-counting CT. *Opt. Express* 28 (17): 25180–25193. https://doi.org/10.1364/OE.400108.

5 Quality Assurance/ Quality Control Considerations

Rad Tech's Guide to Photon Counting Computed Tomography,
First Edition. Euclid Seeram.
© 2025 John Wiley & Sons, Inc. Published 2025 by John Wiley & Sons, Inc.

Introduction

The principles of quality assurance (QA) and quality control (QC) for conventional radiographic imaging systems have been described in detail in the literature [1–5]. For CT systems using EIDs (Chapter 2), QA and QC have been described in detail by the American College of Radiology (ACR) using the ACR CT Accreditation Phantom (CTAP) [6]. The introduction of new CT scanners based on PCDs has raised the question whether the current ACR requirements are suitable to evaluate the special technical features of PCD-CT systems.

The purpose of this chapter is threefold: [1] to provide a general overview of QC with respect to definitions, followed by a brief description of three fundamental steps of QC; [2] to summarize the elements of the ACR manual for QC of CT systems; and [3] to outline essential findings of a major study to establishing a QA program for a PCD-CT imaging system.

What Is Quality Assurance/ Quality Control?

The definitions of QA and QC have been identified in the literature [1–5]. In a nutshell, these definitions reflect that:

- QA addresses the administrative aspects of patient care and quality outcomes. In this regard correct documentation and interpretation of data collected are of significant importance.
- QC is a component of QA and deals with monitoring the technical aspects of the equipment by performing specific tests of important variables that affect not only image

quality but also the radiation dose and with interpretation of the results of the tests.

Specifically, for CT, the ACR defines QA and QC as follows:

- QA "is a comprehensive concept that comprises all of the oversight and management practices developed by the CT imaging team led by the supervising physician ..." [6].
- QC "is an integral part of quality assurance. Quality control is a series of distinct technical procedures that identifies defects or imperfections in a product such that the production process can be altered or corrected to eliminate these defects" [6].

Three Major Components of a Quality Control Program

A QC program consists of three major components, namely, acceptance testing, routine performance, and error correction [1].

1. *Acceptance testing* is the first step of these three activities and ensures that the equipment meets the specifications set by the manufacturers.
2. *Routine performance* refers to the process of conducting the relevant QC tests on the equipment. Furthermore, tests are performed daily, weekly, monthly, semiannually, and annually.
3. *Error correction* is the final step, which means that the equipment fails the test if it does not meet the performance criteria or tolerance limit established for all QC tests, and therefore it must be replaced or repaired to meet tolerance limits.

Performance Criteria

An important characteristic of QC testing is that of *performance criteria*. These criteria for QC test results are stated in terms of *action limits* or *control limits*, which are defined by ± values, that is, the acceptable range of values, as stated in the QC program. Values beyond the limits are rejected and corrective action is required. In this regard, the test must be repeated after consultation with the qualified medical physicist (QMP) and/or QC technologist. For example, when using the ACR CT QC Phantom, the ACR recommends that the quantitative value for the CT number for water should be 0 ± 5 HU, but must be 0 ± 7 HU [7].

The American College of Radiology Quality Control Manual for Computed Tomography

The ACR provides a guidance manual for CT QC tests and state that the manual "provides a minimum set of tests required to ensure that a scanner performs in a consistent manner and yields acceptable images" [7]. Specifically, this manual addresses QC tests for CT scanners based on EIDs.

The manual is organized into three major sections, namely, radiologist's section, radiologic technologist's section, and a QMP's section. Furthermore, each section describes specific responsibilities and technical considerations such as, for example, the QC tests that should be conducted by the technologist and those that should be done by QMP. There are specific tests that are intended for the technologist and for the QMP. For example, tests for the technologist include water CT number and standard deviation (noise), artifact evaluation, wet laser printer QC, a visual checklist, hard copy image QC of dry laser printers, and gray-level performance of CT scanner acquisition display monitors. For the QMP, a representative set of QC tests includes, for example, table travel accuracy, radiation beam width, low-contrast performance, spatial resolution, CT number accuracy, artifact evaluation, CT number uniformity, dosimetry, and CT scanner display calibration.

The format for each test is based on each of the following headings: objectives of the test, frequency of conducting the test, equipment required, test procedure, data interpretation and analysis, precautions and caveats, and corrective action. Furthermore, the manual suggests that the ACR CT Phantom or other manufacturers' CT phantom may be used in conducting the tests.

The American College of Radiology Computed Tomography Phantom

The ACR CT Phantom has been described in the literature [1, 2, 6, 8], and reviewed here in brief. The phantom is shown in Figure 5.1 and consists of four separate modules (Figure 5.1) designed to provide quantitative measures of the required image

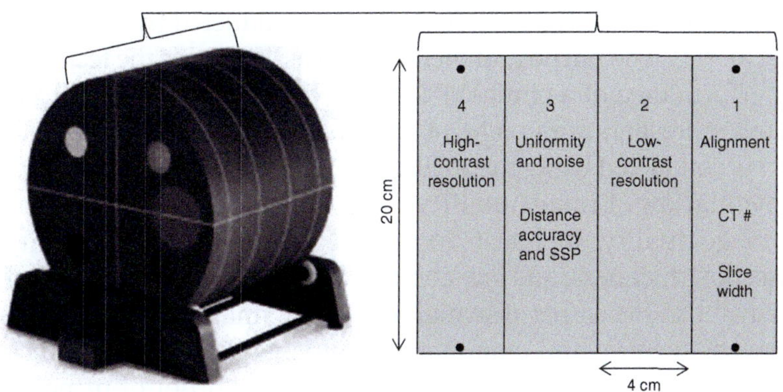

Figure 5.1 The American College of Radiology computed tomography (CT) quality control Accreditation Phantom showing the four modules for the evaluation of standard image quality, such as, for example, CT number accuracy and uniformity, section thickness, and low-contrast and high-contrast resolution.

quality parameters. The phantom is a solid phantom fabricated from a water-equivalent material and made of solid water, a characteristic feature that makes the phantom "a physically stable device that provides reproducible results over time" [6]. The CT scanner parameters that can be examined by the ACR CT Phantom as shown in Figure 5.1 include positioning accuracy, CT number accuracy, slice thickness, low-contrast resolution, high-contrast (spatial) resolution, CT number uniformity, and image noise [6]. For more detailed information on the ACR CT Phantom, the interested reader should refer to references Albus [8], Mansour et al. [6], and Hobson et al. [9].

Establishing a Quality Control Program for a Clinical Photon Counting Detector Computed Tomography System

A technical evaluation of the first PCD-CT Scanner approved by the U.S. FDA [10] for clinical use was conducted by Rajendran et al. [11]. The purpose of their study was "to assess the technical performance of a clinical PCD CT system by using phantoms and representative images of study participants" [11]. The study was conducted using the ACR CTAP and examined quantitative evaluation of image quality, such as evaluation of standard image quality, such as CT number accuracy and uniformity, section thickness, and low-contrast and high-contrast resolution, advanced measures of spatial resolution, image noise and noise power spectra, and quantitative multienergy CT performance. Furthermore, the study also examined a "proof-of-principle study involving participants." The conclusion of this technical evaluation showed that "the first clinical photon-counting detector CT system demonstrated superior spatial resolution, improved noise properties, and better multienergy temporal resolution relative to similarly configured energy-integrating detector CT. Visual correlation of phantom results was shown in humans for four clinical applications" [11].

In yet another study titled "Establishing a Quality Assurance Program for Photon Counting Detector (PCD) CT: Tips and Caveats," Ahmed et al. [12] point out that the special design and functional characteristics of PCDs do not lend themselves to QC procedures designed for CT scanners using EIDs. These characteristics are summarized in Table 5.1. Scan data were reconstructed to generate low-energy threshold (T3D) along with virtual monoenergetic images (VMIs) between 40 and 120 keV.

Table 5.1 Features of PCDs that may limit the direct translation of QC procedures that were designed for conventional CT systems built on EIDs.

Specifically,

PCDs weigh each detected photon the same irrespective of its energy, whereas EIDs weigh the detected photons proportionally to their deposited energy. As a result, PCD-CT generates images with a lower effective energy than their EID-CT counterparts, resulting in different CT numbers for the same materials, even if the acquisition and reconstruction parameters are similar. Therefore, acceptable CT number ranges selected for EID-CT systems may not be valid for PCD-CT systems.

Additionally, PCDs can be manufactured with a smaller form factor than EIDs without a loss of geometric efficiency as they do not need septa materials to prevent visible light from crossing over to neighboring detector pixels. As a result, PCD-CT systems can achieve higher spatial resolution than can EID-CT. Therefore, the range of clinical spatial resolution assessed with conventional phantoms designed for EID-CT may no longer be suitable to characterize certain PCD-CT clinical protocols. Finally, PCD provides intrinsic multienergy information by means of two or more energy thresholds applied to the detected photons. This capability and the need to assess overall detector stability may require changes to the number and frequency of QC tests performed to assess spectral performance.

CT, computed tomography; EID, energy-integrating detector; PCD, photon-counting detector; QC, quality control.
Source: Ahmed et al. [12]/John Wiley & Sons/CC BY 4.0.

A Word About Virtual Monoenergetic Images

VMIs are created through using dual-energy analysis methods, namely, image data–based analysis schematically shown in Figure 5.2 and raw data–based analysis shown in Figure 5.3. While raw data-based analysis involves postprocessing scans before reconstruction, image data-based analysis involves post-processing after "the reconstruction of high- and low-energy images to create various dual-energy CT applications" [13]. Image data–based analysis results in CT artifacts such as beam hardening, motion, and spiral/helical artifacts and are less accurate than scans acquired with the raw data–based approach. These artifacts can be reduced using the raw data–based analysis (as illustrated in Figure 5.4 for beam-hardening artifacts) and results in more accurate attenuation readings. Herein lies one of the

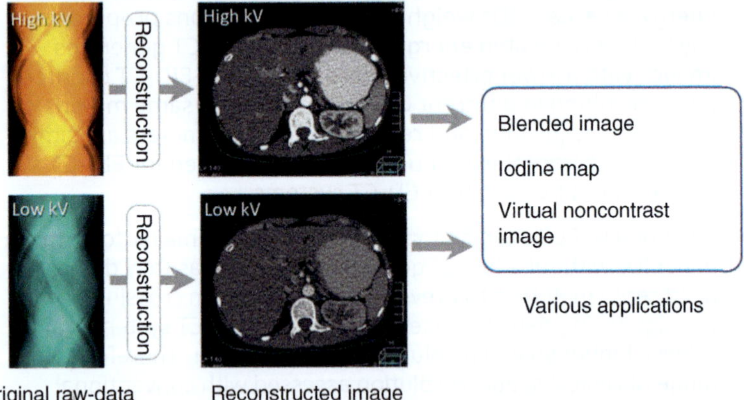

Figure 5.2 Image-based approach for dual-energy computed tomography (CT) analysis. The X-ray paths at high- and low-tube voltages do not need to be perfectly matched. Dual-energy data are processed after the reconstruction of high- and low-energy images and then various applications are created. Dual-energy CT images created by image-based analysis contain various artifacts, for example, beam-hardening, motion, and helical artifacts.
Source: Tatsugami et al. [13]/Springer Nature/CC BY 4.0.

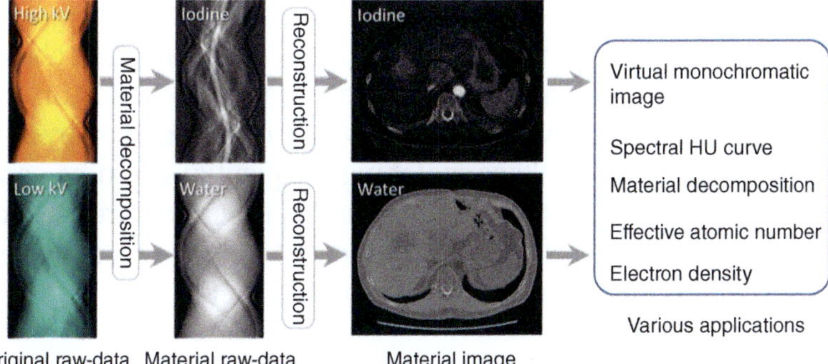

Figure 5.3 Raw data-based approach for dual-energy computed tomography (CT) analysis. The X-ray paths at the high- and low-tube voltages must match exactly. Material raw data are processed directly by material decomposition and then image reconstruction is performed. The obtained CT applications have fewer beam-hardening effects and artifacts related to the CT reconstruction kernel than do image-based analysis.

Source: Tatsugami et al. [13]/Springer Nature/CC BY 4.0.

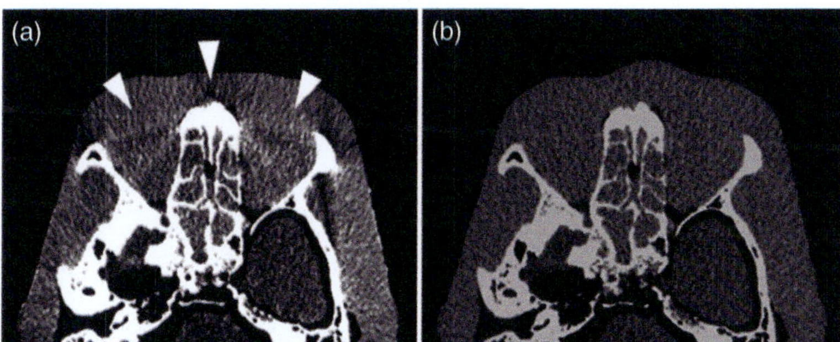

Figure 5.4 Computed tomography (CT) image processed with image-based analysis (a) and raw data-based analysis (b). In image-based analysis, beam-hardening artifacts from facial bones degrade the image quality (arrowheads). As the CT image processed with raw data-based analysis rather than image-based analysis exhibits lower beam-hardening artifacts, the acquired CT number would be accurate.

Source: Tatsugami et al. [13]/Springer Nature/CC BY 4.0.

major advantages of virtual monochromatic dual-energy CT image analysis [13]. The final point about VMIs is that "the choice between raw data– and image-based analysis depends on the dual-energy CT hardware. Currently, raw data–based analysis is used with fast tube-voltage switching-, sequential scanning-, and dual-layer detector systems. Dual-source CT scanners are used for image-based analysis" [13]. Further details of these methods are described by Tatsugami et al. [13] and Liang et al. [14].

QC Testing

Using the ACR CTAP and recommendations, they conducted the following QC tests:

1. The daily CT QC procedure be performed by the technologist prior to the first clinical scan of the day "to (a) ensure stable calibration of CT numbers relative to water, (b) ensure stable image noise, and (c) identify any image artifacts before patient scanning."
2. The annual CT equipment performance evaluation for CT number linearity at all available tube potentials (see Ahmed et al. [12] for details) and slice thickness, low-contrast detectability, spatial uniformity, and high-contrast spatial resolution.

Results

The results for the daily CT QC images are shown in Figure 5.5. While the top row of images shows a clear center-dot artifact, the bottom row of images shows a significant reduction of the artifact after detector replacement [12]. On the other hand, the results for the annual CT equipment performance evaluation are summarized in Table 5.2. Furthermore, Ahmed et al. [12] performed additional tests such as the spatial resolution of PCD-CT's ultra-high-resolution (UHR) mode using the modulation

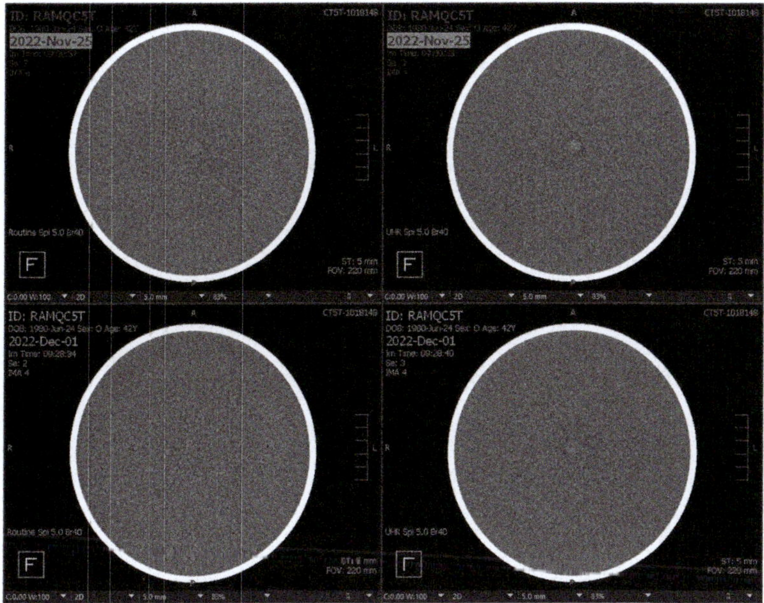

Figure 5.5 Daily computed tomography (CT) quality control images from the photon-counting detector CT system. Top row, initial data acquired in spiral mode with the standard (144×04 mm; left) and ultra-high resolution (UHR) (120×0.2 mm; right) detector configuration. Hyperdense artifact at the isocenter was noted, most prominent in the UHR mode, which contributed to the decision to replace detector modules during a scheduled system upgrade the following day. Bottom row, the same data acquired after the detector module replacement showed the artifact was strongly decreased.

Source: Ahmed et al. [12]/John Wiley & Sons/CC BY 4.0.

transfer function (MTF) curve [1], and an iodine map using "a multi-energy CT phantom (40×30 cm [2]; Sun Nuclear) containing four solid inserts with iodine concentrations of 2, 5, 10, and 15 mg L/cc and reconstructing an iodine map along with VMIs between 40 and 120 keV" [12].

The results showed that the limiting resolution of the PDC operating in the UHR mode is about 40 lp/cm as shown in Figure 5.6. Recall that the limiting resolution is the spatial

Table 5.2 A summary of the results of the annual CT equipment performance evaluation.

Module 1	Modules 2 and 3	Module 4
CT number linearity	**Low contrast detectability and spatial uniformity, respectively**	**High-contrast spatial resolution**
The first module of the ACR CTAP includes five inserts (water, air, polyethylene, acrylic, and bone) and their CT numbers should fall within a prescribed range for a 120-kV scan. For the EID-CT data, all measurements were within the limits of the 120-kV single-energy acquisitions. For the PCD-CT data, the measured CT number for the bone insert was 1001 HU at 120 kV when using T3D images, which exceeds the upper limit of 970 HU in the ACR manual. On the other hand, all measurements were within the prescribed limits for the 70 keV VMI we used on the four routine clinical protocols. Other VMI reconstructions were also tested between 40 and 120 keV in steps of 10 keV/step, but only the 70 keV reconstruction was within limits for all inserts.	There were no substantial differences between EID-CT and PCD-CT on the second and third modules of the ACR CTAP. In the figure below, images of the central slice are shown for both modules and the EID-CT and PCD-CT scanners, using the routine adult head protocol. The performance is similar between the two systems, albeit the lower noise in the PCD-CT images at matched spatial resolution (reconstruction kernel) allows for increased detectability of low-contrast objects, such as the 5- and 4-mm inserts. 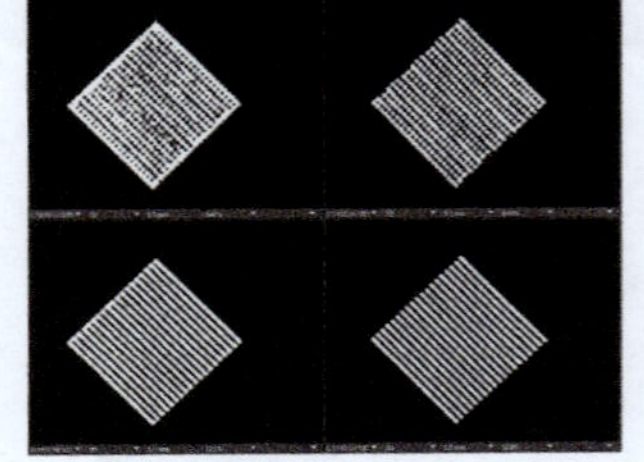	The figure below shows a close-up view of the highest resolution insert (12 lp/cm) for module 4 of the ACR CTAP phantom scanned on EID-CT and PCD-CT using the routine adult head protocol. Both the EID-CT and PCD-CT were able to resolve this insert with the typical bone reconstruction kernel, especially if higher resolution matrices (>512) are available. However, the PCD-CT has an additional ultra-high-resolution mode that can achieve even greater resolutions that significantly exceed the ACR CTAP. 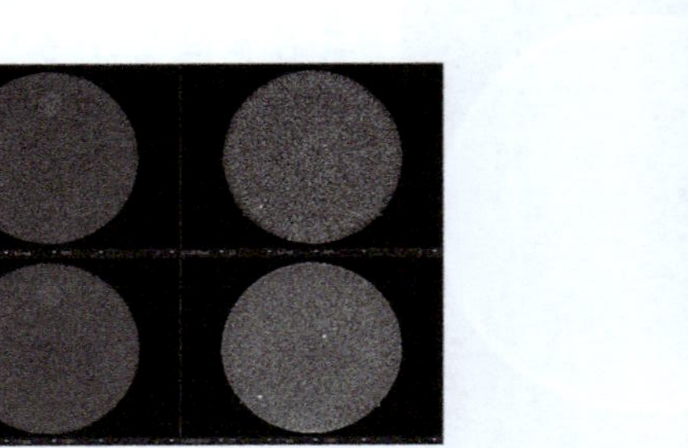

ACR, American College of Radiology; CT, computed tomography; CTAP, CT Accreditation Phantom; EID, energy-integrating detector; HU, Hounsfield units; PCD, photon-counting detector; VMI, virtual monoenergetic image.
Source: Ahmed et al. [12]/John Wiley & Sons/CC BY 4.0.

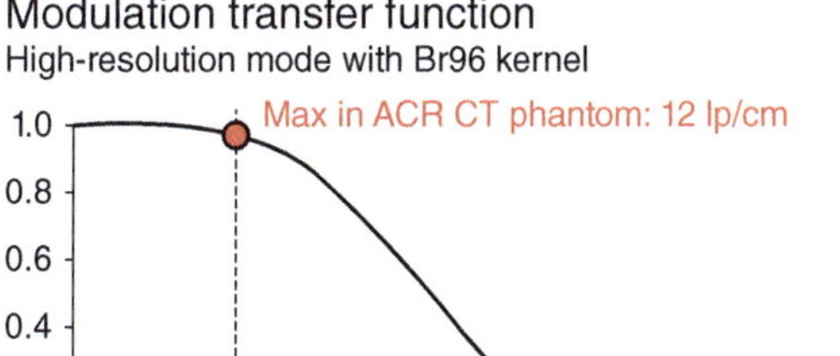

Figure 5.6 The modulation transfer function measured from the photon-counting detector computed tomography (PCD-CT) using the ultra-high-resolution mode with a sharp kernel. The limiting resolution is near 40 lp/cm, which is far greater than the maximum resolution of 12 lp/cm in the American College of Radiology CT phantom.

Source: Ahmed et al. [12]/John Wiley & Sons/CC BY 4.0.

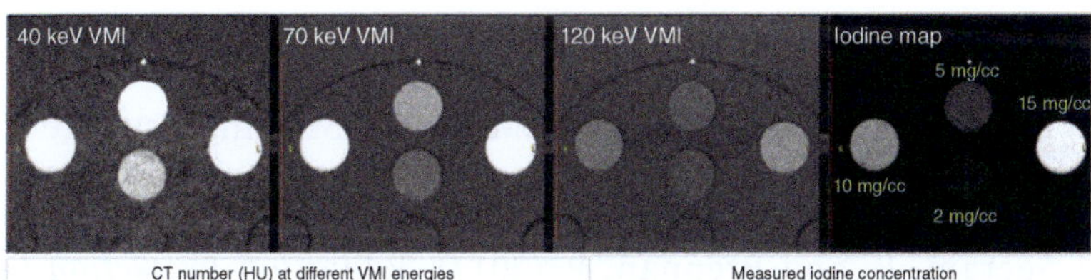

Figure 5.7 Sample images of the multienergy phantom (see text) at different VMIs along with the iodine map. The iodine concentration of the four inserts is overlaid on the iodine map. The measured computed tomography number in each insert was in good agreement (3.8% mean percent error) with the reference values provided by the phantom manufacturer. HU, Hounsfield units; VMI, virtual monoenergetic image.

Source: Ahmed et al. [12]/John Wiley & Sons/CC BY 4.0.

frequency at an MTF equal to 0.1 [1]. Furthermore, sample images of the multienergy phantom at different VMIs along with the iodine map is shown in (Figure 5.7). The iodine concentration of the four inserts is overlaid on the iodine map, and the measured CT number in each insert was in good agreement

(3.8% mean percent error) with the reference values provided by the phantom manufacturer [12].

In the article on establishing a QC program for PCCT, Ahmed et al. [12] conclude that "while the ACR CTAP phantom has been routinely used in CT quality control, precautions need to be taken in its uses on clinical PCD-CT and protocols/parameters should be properly selected to meet current accreditation requirements. For quality control purposes, VMIs (e.g., 70 keV) may be more suitable than energy-thresholded 120-kV images. Additional evaluations such as MTF measurements and multi-energy scans are also recommended to fully evaluate scanner performance" [12].

References

1 Bushong, S. (2023). *Radiologic Science for Technologists*, 12e. St Louis, MO: Elsevier.
2 Seeram, E. (2019). *Digital Radiography: Physical Principles, and Quality Control*, 2e. Springer Nature Singapore Pte Ltd.
3 Katzman, G.L. and Paushter, D.M. (2016). Building a culture of continuous quality improvement in an academic radiology department. *J. Am. Coll. Radiol.* 13 (4): 453–460.
4 Seeram, E. and Brennan, P. (2017). *Radiation Protection in Diagnostic Imaging*. Burlington, MA: Jones and Bartlett Learning.
5 AAPM. Report no. (2006). *93 Acceptance Testing and Quality Control of Photostimulable Storage Phosphor Imaging Systems Report of AAPM Task Group 10*. College Park, MD: AAPM.
6 Mansour, Z., Mokhtar, A., Sarhan, A. et al. (2016). Quality control of CT image using American College of Radiology (ACR) phantom. *Egypt. J. Radiol. Nucl. Med.* 47 (4): 1665–1167. https://doi.org/10.1016/j.ejrnm.2016.08.016.
7 American College of Radiology (ACR) (2017). Computed tomography manual. https://www.acr.org/-/media/ACR/Files/Clinical-Resources/QC-Manuals/CT_QCManual.pdf (accessed November 2024).

8 Albus, K. (2024). Phantom overview: CT (Revised 1 March 2024). `https://accreditationsupport.acr.org/support/solutions/articles/11000053945-phantom-overview-ct-revised-1-3-2024` (accessed November 2024).

9 Hobson, M.A., Soisson, E.T., Davis, S.D., and Parker, W. (2014). Using the ACR CT accreditation phantom for routine image quality assurance on both CT and CBCT imaging systems in a radiotherapy environment. *J. Appl. Clin. Med. Phys.* 15 (4): 4835. `https://doi.org/10.1120/jacmp.v15i4.4835`. Erratum in: J. Appl. Clin. Med. Phys. 2014 Nov 08;15(6):5 228. 10.1120/jacmp.v15i6.5228. PMID: 25207412; PMCID: PMC5875525.

10 US Food and Drug Administration (2022). FDA clears first major imaging device advancement for computed tomography in nearly a decade. `https://www.fda.gov/news-events/press-announcements/fda-clears-first-major-imaging-device-advancement-computed-tomography-nearly-decade` (accessed 1 November 2022).

11 Rajendran, K., Petersilka, M., Henning, A. et al. (2022). First clinical photon counting-detector CT system: technical evaluation. *Radiology* 303 (1): 130.

12 Ahmed, Z., Ferrero, A., Ren, L. et al. (2023). Establishing a quality assurance program for photon counting detector (PCD) CT: tips and caveats. *J. Appl. Clin. Med. Phys.* 24: e14074. `https://doi.org/10.1002/acm2.14074`.

13 Tatsugami, F., Higaki, T., Nakamura, Y. et al. (2022). Dual-energy CT: minimal essentials for radiologists. *Jpn. J. Radiol.* 40: 547–559. `https://doi.org/10.1007/s11604-021-01233-2`.

14 Liang, H., Zhou, Y., Zheng, Q. et al. (2022). Dual-energy CT with virtual monoenergetic images and iodine maps improves tumor conspicuity in patients with pancreatic ductal adenocarcinoma. *Insights Imaging* 13: 153. `https://doi.org/10.1186/s13244-022-01297-2`.

6

Clinical Applications of Photon-Counting Computed Tomography: A Brief Overview

Chapter at a Glance

Rad Tech's Guide to Photon Counting Computed Tomography,
First Edition. Euclid Seeram.
© 2025 John Wiley & Sons, Inc. Published 2025 by John Wiley & Sons, Inc.

Introduction

The advantages of PCCT compared with EID-CT have been discussed in Chapter 4. In summary, these benefits include improved spatial resolution and higher dose efficiency resulting in reduced dose to patients and hence enabling low-dose CT imaging, reduction of electronic noise, reduction of artifacts, and multienergy CT imaging. Table 6.1 shows the clinical applications that would benefit significantly from the specific advantages of PCCT.

An important literature review of clinical applications is provided by Tortora et al. [2] for head and neck, temporal bone, breast, cardiovascular, abdominal, and musculoskeletal imaging. In a similar vein, other reviews of clinical applications are provided by several authors [1, 3–8]. Furthermore, other reviews have focussed on anatomical areas such as the chest [9],

Table 6.1 The advantages of photon-counting CT linked to their clinical applications.

Advantages	Physical properties	Clinical applications
High spatial resolution	1. Directly measuring the X-ray absorption of a single photon without adding electronic noise from the detectors 2. More accurate determination of photon path resulting in higher spatial resolution 3. Using smaller pixels to improve resolution further	■ Small lesion detection in oncology ■ Improved visualization of small vessels in neuroimaging ■ Improved detection of bone micro-fractures ■ Improved visualization of small structures such as coronary arteries, small lung nodules, and fine bony structures

Table 6.1 (Continued)

Advantages	Physical properties	Clinical applications
Improved iodine signal	1. Separating the K-edge signals of iodine from the polychromatic spectrum of X-rays 2. Measuring the energy of each X-ray photon to calculate the iodine concentration	■ Accurate and precise measurement of iodine concentration in organs, especially in the liver and pancreas ■ Improved detection of iodine-based contrast agents in CT angiography
Radiation dose optimization	1. Using a lower tube current to reduce radiation dose 2. Using a higher energy threshold to avoid unnecessary low-energy photons	■ Reduced radiation exposure for pediatric, young adult patients, and patients with cancer with continuous follow-up ■ Enhanced monitoring of patient's radiation exposure over time ■ Improved safety for repeat imaging exams
Artifact reduction	1. Reducing beam-hardening artifacts by separating the polychromatic X-ray beam into different energy bins. 2. Reducing metal artifacts by separating photons based on energy and material composition	■ Reduced metal artifacts in orthopedic implants and dental fillings ■ Improved image quality in patients with high body mass index ■ Improved visualization of complex anatomy in head and neck imaging

(Continued)

Table 6.1 (Continued)

Advantages	Physical properties	Clinical applications
Multienergy imaging	1. Separating photons based on their energy to distinguish between different tissue types 2. Allowing for the quantification of tissue composition and characterization	■ Improved differentiation between contrast enhancement and hemorrhage in acute stroke imaging ■ Improved detection and characterization of gout in musculoskeletal imaging ■ Improved treatment planning and monitoring for conditions such as joint replacement, organ transplant, and dental implants

CT, computed tomography.
Source: Reproduced from Wu et al. [1]/with permission of Elsevier.

temporal bone [10], abdomen [11], and spine [12] and on cardiovascular diseases [13] and neurovascular imaging [14].

This chapter will provide a narrative review of PCCT applications in imaging the chest, temporal bone, abdomen, cardiovascular diseases, and musculoskeletal imaging. It is not within the scope of this chapter to explore all clinical applications of PCCT. Therefore, the reader must refer to the full articles for more details of these applications.

Clinical Applications of Photon-Counting Computed Tomography

It is important to note here that the applications highlighted in the following sections compare the imaging performance of PCCT with EID CT in demonstrating not only anatomical features but also various pathologies. It is also not within the scope of this chapter to describe the various methodologies of these research studies. Interested readers should refer to the original studies appropriately cited in the references.

Chest Imaging

The chest is the most common anatomical area imaged in the radiology department using diagnostic X-rays, to show "normal anatomy and variants ... and pathology of the heart, mediastinum, lungs and pleura, chest wall and abdomen" [15].

As discussed by Tortora et al. [2], the advantage of high spatial resolution has resulted in PCCT showing "a more precise assessment of nodules and the smallest pulmonary structures such as the terminal divisions of the bronchial tree and the interstitium" [2]. Furthermore, Tortora et al. [2] cited various studies reporting that PCCT shows improved clarity of solitary pulmonary nodules, pulmonary parenchyma, interstitial lung disease, bronchiectasis, and so forth [2].

Temporal Bone Imaging

The spatial resolution advantage of PCCT has been shown to be beneficial in temporal bone imaging. The temporal bone "contains the middle and inner portions of the ear, and is crossed by the majority of the cranial nerves. The lower portion of the bone articulates with the mandible, forming the temporomandibular joint of the jaw" [16]. It also contains very tiny structures such as the ossicles [16]. PCCT spatial resolution advantage is extremely useful to show details of these structures with good clarity.

The clinical applications of PCCT in temporal bone imaging is well documented in the literature by several investigators [10, 17–21]. The general conclusions of these studies show that PCCT provides improved image quality of the fine structures of the temporal bone compared with EID-CT scanners. Examples of this image comparison are shown in Figure 6.1 for the tegmen tympani and Figure 6.2 for the ossicles in the inner ear.

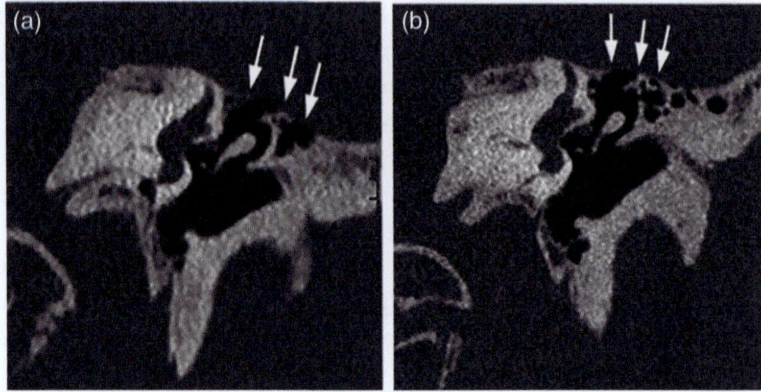

Figure 6.1 A comparison of the image quality of the tegmen tympani (arrows) obtained with an energy-integrating detector computed tomography scanner (a) and a photon-counting computed tomography scanner (b). It is clear that image (b) shows this specific anatomy much better that image (a).

Source: Reproduced with permission from Hermans et al. [17]/Springer Nature/CC BY 4.0.

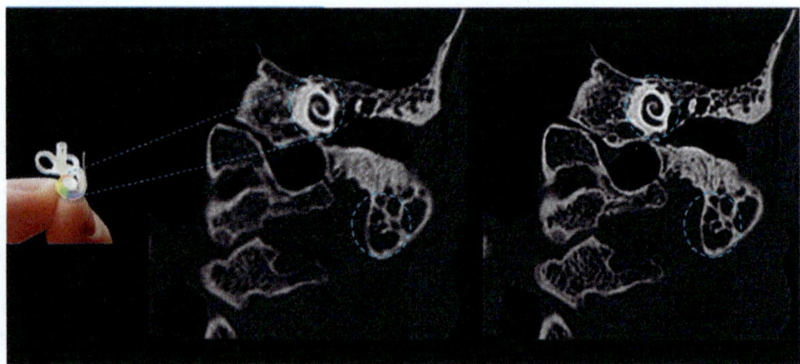

Figure 6.2 Photon-counting computed tomography imaging shows excellent spatial resolution of the ossicles of the inner ear.

Source: Courtesy of NeuroLogica.

Abdominal Imaging

The anatomy and various pathologies of the abdomen are reviewed in Radiology Cafe [22], and several clinical applications of PCCT in imaging the abdomen have been described in the literature [7, 11, 23–25].

Pourmorteza et al. [23] reported the first PCCT imaging of humans in an article titled "Abdominal Imaging with Contrast-Enhanced Photon-Counting CT: First Human Experience." The overall goal of their study was to assess a prototype PCCT scanner in imaging of the human abdomen, compared with an EID CT scanner. The investigators concluded that there was no statistically significant difference between PCCT and EID-CT in imaging the abdomen, and the spectral information from PCCT is useful in material decomposition [23]. Onishi et al. [11] showed that the PCCT advantages of high CNR, high spatial resolution, and the creation of VMIs may result in improved visualization of images of the liver, pancreas, and vascular anatomical structures of the abdomen, at reduced radiation doses to patients.

The high CNR advantage enables improved visualization of small or low-contrast lesions as illustrated in Figure 6.3, together with the lower-radiation-dose PCCT ($CTDI_{vol}$: 7.5 mGy) than with conventional CT (11.9 mGy) [11]. Furthermore, the advantage of VMIs is shown in Figure 6.4, where VMIs at lower keV settings result in higher contrast "between the liver lesion and the liver parenchyma" [11]. In addition, the high spatial resolution of PCCT makes this imaging modality very useful in vascular imaging such as in CT angiography (CTA), as demonstrated in Figure 6.5a, where "in this case, hepatocellular carcinoma was treated by transarterial chemoembolization, and celiac angiography was also performed during the procedure Figure 6.5b. CT angiography adequately delineated the hepatic artery to the periphery, which may facilitate selective catheter insertion into the hepatic artery branches" [26].

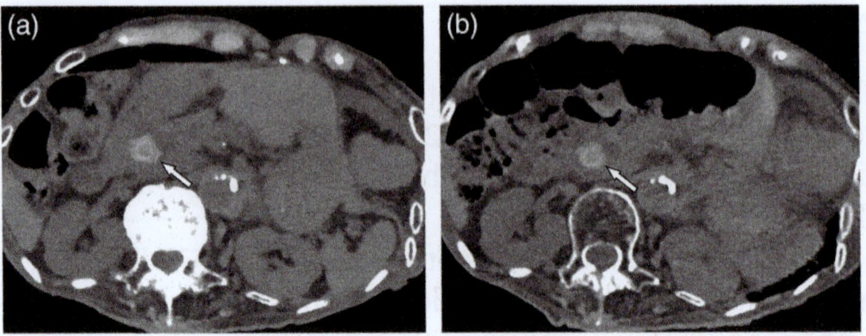

Figure 6.3 Noncontrast abdominal computed tomography (CT) images of a patient with choledocholithiasis showed that the layered calcified stone in the common bile duct (arrows) is visualized more precisely with photon-counting CT (a) than with conventional dual-source CT (single-energy mode) (b). The radiation dose was lower with photon-counting CT (CTDI$_{vol}$ 7.5 mGy) than with conventional CT (11.9 mGy).

Source: Reproduced with permission from Onishi et al. [11]/Springer Nature/CC BY 4.0.

Additional studies on the usefulness of PCCT in imaging the abdomen are ones by Khanungwanitku et al. [7], Schwartz et al. [24], and Graafen et al. [25] While the study by Khanungwanitku et al. [7] showed several advantages in liver disease assessment, differentiation between adrenal and renal masses, as well as dose optimization for patients who are subject to repeat examinations, the study of Schwartz et al. [24] explored PCCT imaging of cystic lesions, sources of bleeding, and cancers. Finally, the study by Graafen et al. [25] examined the use of PCCT in imaging arterial phase abdominal scans. They showed that VMIs taken at low keV provides better quality of "arterial phase oncological imaging compared with EID-CT" [25].

Musculoskeletal Imaging

In order to appreciate the clinical applications of PCCT details of the anatomy and physiology of the musculoskeletal system, it is important to have a good understanding of the anatomy

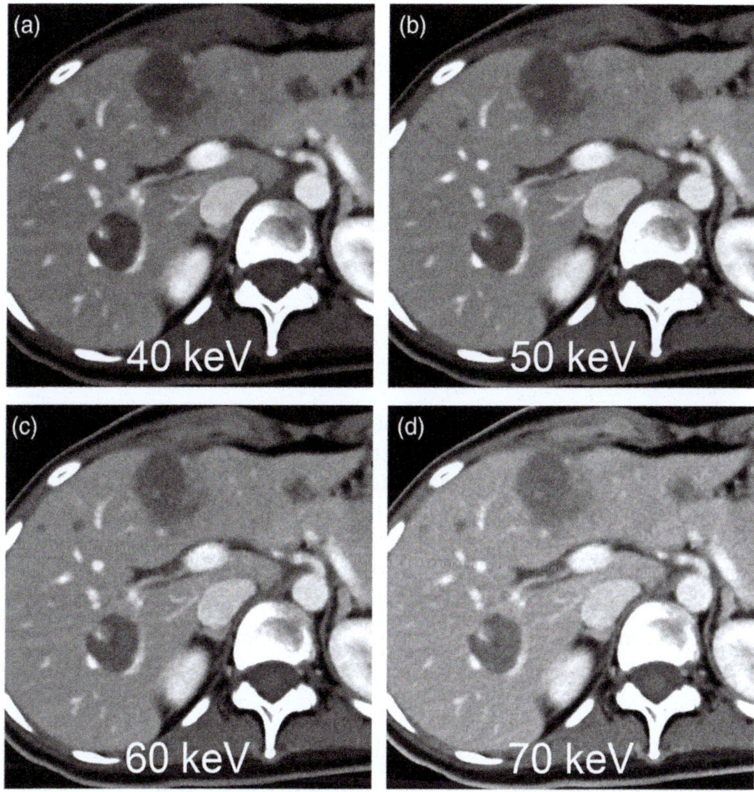

Figure 6.4 Using a photon-counting detector, virtual monochromatic images of any energy level from 40 to 190 keV can be generated from 120 kVp single-energy raw data. The lower the keV setting of the virtual monochromatic image, the higher the contrast between the liver lesion and the liver parenchyma.

Source: Reproduced with permission from Onishi et al. [11]/Springer Nature/CC BY 4.0.

and physiology of this system. A good review is provided by Sendic [27]. Furthermore, this system can also be reviewed in any good anatomy and physiology textbook. It is important that the imaging system demonstrates, for example, trabecular details of the bones as well as details of the muscles.

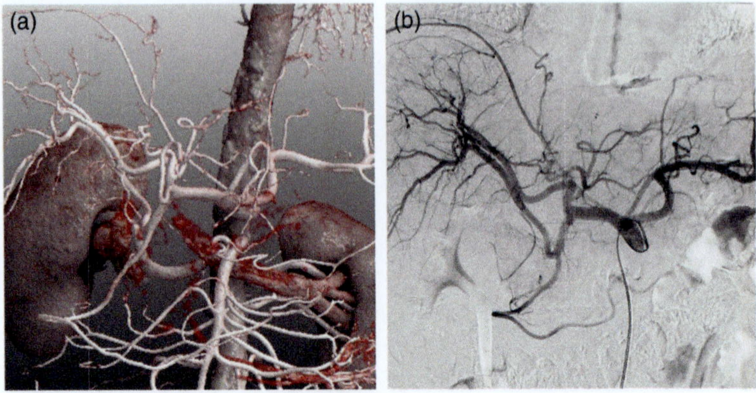

Figure 6.5 Photon-counting computed tomography (CT) is also excellent for CT angiography (a) because of its superior spatial resolution. In this case, hepatocellular carcinoma was treated by transarterial chemoembolization, and celiac angiography was also performed during the procedure (b). CT angiography adequately delineated the hepatic artery to the periphery, which may facilitate selective catheter insertion into the hepatic artery branches.

Source: Reproduced with permission from Onishi et al. [11]/Springer Nature/CC BY 4.0.

Several articles have focussed on the use of PCCT in imaging the musculoskeletal system such as, for example, those by Mourad et al. [28], Grunz et al. [29], Bette et al. [30], Grunz et al. [31], Baffour et al. [32], and Eibschutz et al. [33] While the details of these studies are beyond the scope of this book, the following are key takeaways:

- Mourad et al. [28], for example, showed that the "high-spatial resolution imaging for the assessment of bone and crystal deposits, low-dose applications such as whole-body CT, as well as spectral imaging applications including the characterization of crystal deposits and imaging of metal hardware" [28]. The gains in spatial resolution and metal artifact reduction are shown in Figures 6.6, 6.7 and 6.8, respectively.

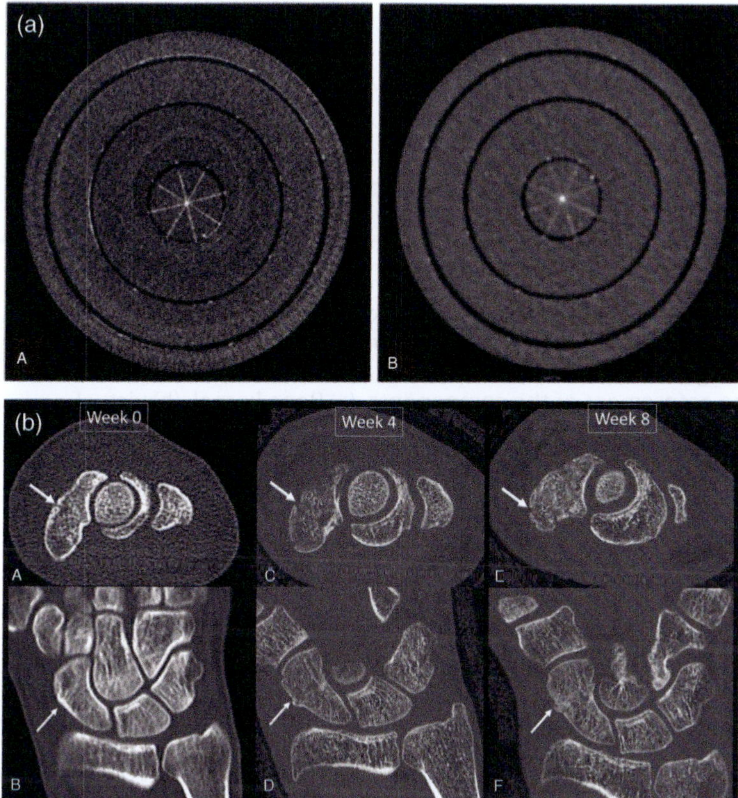

Figure 6.6 Improved spatial resolution between photon-counting detector computed tomography (PCD-CT) (a) and energy-integrating detector dual-energy computed tomography (EID-DECT) (b) Improved spatial resolution between an EID-DECT (A, B) and clinical PCD-CT (C-F) is shown in (b).

Source: Reproduced with permission from Mourad et al. [28]/Springer Nature/CC BY 4.0.

- Baffour et al. [32] showed that improved spatial resolution of PCCT provided better cortical and trabecular detail, as well as skeletal abnormalities, lytic lesions, fractures, and mineralized tumor matrix.

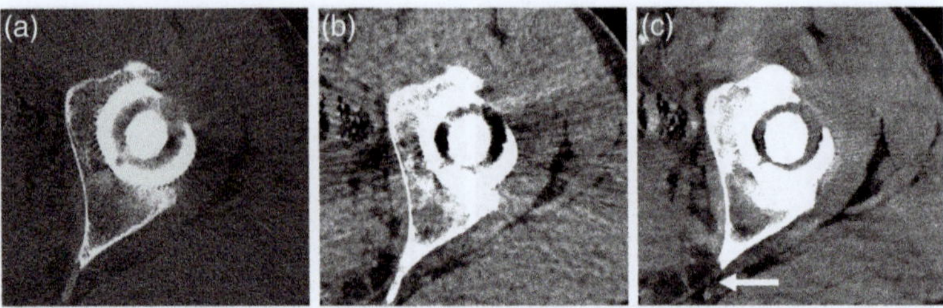

Figure 6.7 Metal artifact reduction: transverse reformats of photon-counting detector computed tomography of a left total hip replacement acquired at 140 kVp with tin filtration, and reconstructed using different parameters, which affect the metal artifacts and the assessment of the components. (a) Bone kernel, (b) virtual monoenergetic image (120 keV) with soft tissue kernel, and (c) virtual monoenergetic image (120 keV) with soft tissue kernel and iterative metal artifact reduction algorithm (same window level as in (b)).

Source: Reproduced with permission from Mourad et al. [28]/Springer Nature/CC BY 4.0.

- A key point reported by Bette et al. [30] notes that "with its ability to routinely acquire spectral data, PCD-CT scans allow for material classification, such as detecting urate crystals in suspected gout or visualizing bone marrow edema, potentially reducing reliance on MRI in certain cases" [30].
- Eibschutz et al. [33] showed that "spectral CT has a considerable role in improving the diagnosis, characterization, and treatment of gout, inflammatory arthropathies, degenerative disc disease, osteoporosis, occult fractures, malignancies, ligamentous injuries, and other bone-marrow pathologies" [28].

The evidence identified in the aforementioned studies regarding the fact that PCCT provides excellent spatial resolution, metal artifact reduction, and material decomposition, Gruntz et al. [29] stress that "many musculoskeletal-specific PCD-CT applications are still in a rather preliminary form or not

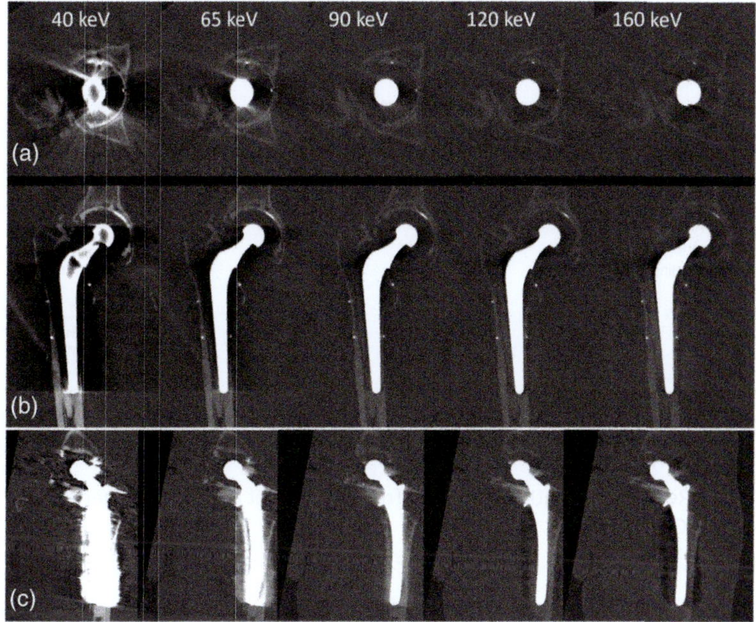

Figure 6.8 Photon-counting detector computed tomography generates virtual monoenergetic images that range from 40 to 160 keV, progressively reducing metal artifacts around total hip replacements and allowing for improved evaluation of the metal–bone interface and surrounding structures.

Source: Reproduced with permission from Mourad et al. [28]/Springer Nature/CC BY 4.0.

yet available for standard clinical routine, hence further studies are necessary to identify more 'game changers' for MSK patient care" [29].

Cardiovascular Imaging

The use of PCCT in cardiac imaging is illustrated in Figure 6.9, which shows that the advantages of improved spatial resolution, artifact reduction, and inherent spectral imaging of PCCT have provided not only improved coronary artery assessment and

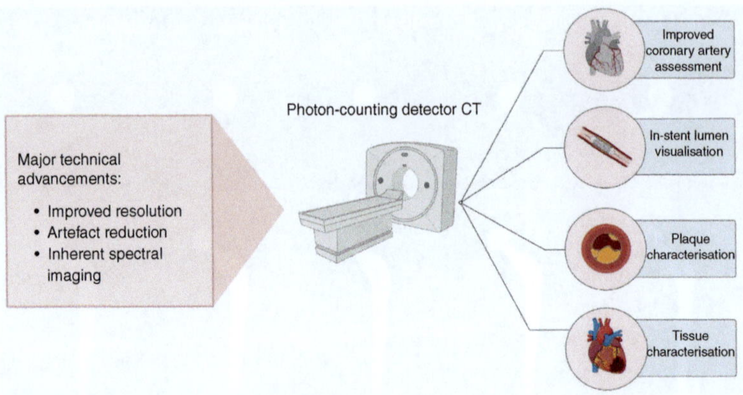

Figure 6.9 The use of photon-counting computed tomography in cardiac imaging.

Source: Reproduced with permission from Sharma et al. [34]/Springer Nature/CC BY 4.0.

in-stent lumen visualization, but also plaque characterization and tissue characterization [34].

The cardiovascular applications of PCCT have been reviewed by several investigators such as Meloni et al. [35], Lacaita et al. [36], Flohr [37], Meloni et al. [13], and Meloni et al. [38], to mention only but a few. The article by Meloni et al. [35] is titled "Cardiovascular Applications of Photon-Counting CT Technology: A Revolutionary New Diagnostic Step." This article first provides a summary of the applications and the main advantages of PCCT in cardiovascular imaging, as shown in Table 6.2. Cardiac/coronary PCCT examples of normal coronary arteries, cardiac/coronary PCCT examples of coronary arteries with standard versus ultra-high spatial resolution, and cardiac/coronary PCCT example of a significant stenosis of proximal left anterior descending coronary artery are shown in Figures 6.10 and 6.11, respectively. Subsequently, they discuss the notion that PCCT "can support the study of myocardial blood perfusion and enable enhanced tissue characterization and

Table 6.2 Cardiovascular applications of photon-counting CT.

- Improved visualization of coronary plaques and patent lumen over conventional CT
- Superior accuracy in the quantification of luminal stenosis across all plaque types compared with conventional CT
- Improved accuracy in coronary artery calcium quantification compared with conventional CT
- Improved detection of coronary calcium even at a reduced radiation dose compared with conventional CT
- Anatomic assessment of plaque composition: differentiation among calcified, fibrous, and lipid-rich plaques and identification of features such as thinning of the fibrous cap or presence of intraplaque hemorrhage
- Potential capability to provide information about the biological activity within the coronary plaque, such as inflammation or neovascularization
- Better visualization of the stent lumen compared with conventional CT
- Improved detection of in-stent restenosis compared with conventional CT
- Quantification of myocardial extracellular volume at a low radiation dose
- Accurate delineation of myocardial scar achieved thanks to the excellent contrast between infarcted myocardium, remote myocardium, and left ventricular blood pool
- Detection of myocardial perfusion defects
- Improved extraction myocardial radiomics features compared with conventional CT
- Accurate quantification of epicardial adipose tissue volume and assessment of pericoronary adipose tissue attenuation
- Reduction in the volume of iodine-based contrast media in coronary CT angiography without compromising the diagnostic image quality

CT, computed tomography.
Source: Adapted from Cardiovascular Applications of Photon-Counting CT Technology.

the identification of contrast agents, in a manner that was previously unattainable" [35].

Other studies identified earlier have focussed on coronary imaging [13, 37]. Last but not least, Lacaita et al. [36] have argued

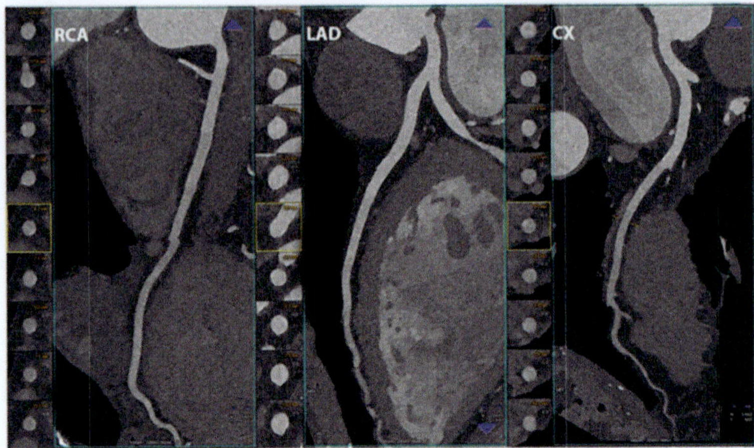

Figure 6.10 Cardiac/coronary photon-counting computed tomography examples of normal coronary arteries, right coronary artery (RCA), the left anterior descending coronary artery (LAD), and for the left circumflex artery (CX).

Source: Reproduced with permission from Meloni et al. [35]/MDPI/CC BY 4.0.

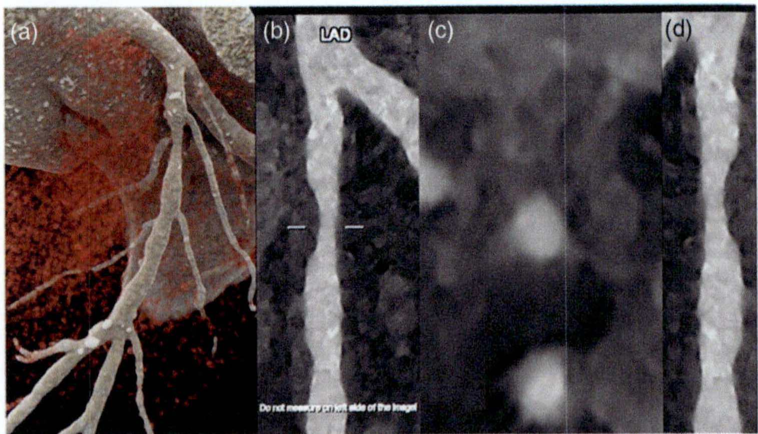

Figure 6.11 Cardiac/coronary photon-counting computed tomography example of a significant stenosis of proximal left anterior descending coronary artery.

Source: Reproduced with permission from Meloni et al. [35]/MDPI/CC BY 4.0.

that "PCD-CT has yet led to a true step-change and significant progress in cardiovascular imaging" [36]. For further details, readers must refer to the full articles as provided in the reference section of this chapter. PCCT has been hailed as the new generation of CT scanners and as such provides "a revolutionary new diagnostic step" [35].

Conclusion

The advantages of PCCT scanners using its special PCD characteristics (Chapter 3) have provided improved clinical information compared with energy-resolving detectors of conventional CT scanners.

References

1 Wu, Y., Ye, Z., Chen, J. et al. (2023). Photon counting CT: technical principles, clinical applications, and future prospects. *Acad. Radiol.* 30 (10): 2362–2382. https://doi.org/10.1016/j.acra.2023.05.029.

2 Tortora, M., Gemini, L., D'Iglio, I. et al. (2022). Spectral photon-counting computed tomography: a review on technical principles and clinical applications. *J. Imaging* 8: 112. https://doi.org/10.3390/jimaging8040112.

3 Rajiah, P., Parakh, A., Kay, F. et al. (2020). Update on multienergy CT: physics, principles, and applications. *RadioGraphics* 40: 1284–1308.

4 Willemink, M.J., Persson, M., Pourmorteza, A. et al. (2018). Photon-counting CT: technical principles and clinical prospects. *Radiology* 289 (2): 293–312.

5 Leng, S., Bruesewitz, M., Tao, S. et al. (2019). Photon-counting detector CT: system design and clinical applications of an emerging technology. *RadioGraphics* 39 (3): 729–743.

6 McCollough, C.H., Rajendran, K., Baffour, F.I. et al. (2023). Clinical applications of photon counting detector CT. *Eur. Radiol.* 33: 5309–5320. https://doi.org/10.1007/s00330-023-09596-y.

7 Khanungwanitkul, K., Sliwicka, O., and Schwartz, F.R. (2024). Abdominal applications of photon-counting CT. *Br. J. Radiol.* tqae206: https://doi.org/10.1093/bjr/tqae206.

8 Hsieh, S.S., Leng, S., Rajendran, K. et al. (2021). Photon counting CT: clinical applications and future developments. *IEEE Trans. Radiat. Plasma Med. Sci.* 5 (4): 441–452. https://doi.org/10.1109/TRPMS.2020.302021.

9 Si-Mohamed, S.A., Miailhes, J., Rodesch, P.-A. et al. (2021). Spectral photon-counting CT technology in chest imaging. *J. Clin. Med.* 10 (24): 5757. https://doi.org/10.3390/jcm1024575.

10 Zhou, W., Lane, L.L., Carlson, M.L. et al. (2018). Comparison of a photon-counting-detector ct with an energy-integrating-detector CT for temporal bone imaging: a cadaveric study. *AJNR Am. J. Neuroradiol.* 39 (9): 1733–1738.

11 Onishi, H., Tsuboyama, T., Nakamoto, A. et al. (2024). Photon-counting CT: technical features and clinical impact on abdominal imaging. *Abdom. Radiol* 49: 4383–4399. https://doi.org/10.1007/s00261-024-04414-5.

12 Rau, A., Straehle, J., Stein, T. et al. (2023 Aug). Photon-counting computed tomography (PC-CT) of the spine: impact on diagnostic confidence and radiation dose. *Eur. Radiol.* 33 (8): 5578–5586. https://doi.org/10.1007/s00330-023-09511-5.

13 Meloni, A., Maffei, E., Clemente, A. et al. (2024). Spectral photon-counting computed tomography: technical principles and applications in the assessment of cardiovascular diseases. *J. Clin. Med.* 13: 2359. https://doi.org/10.3390/jcm13082359.

14 Madhavan, A.A., Bathla, G., Benson, J.C. et al. (2024). High yield clinical applications for photon counting CT in neurovascular imaging. *Br. J. Radiol.* 97 (1157): 894–901. https://doi.org/10.1093/bjr/tqae058.

15 Smithuis, R. and van Delden, O. (2025). Chest X-ray - basic interpretation. Radiology assistant. https://radiologyassistant.nl/chest/chest-x-ray/basic-interpretation (accessed February 2025).

16 Jones, O. (2025). The temporal bone. https://teachmeanatomy.info/head/osteology/temporal-bone/ (accessed February 2025).

17 Hermans, R., Boomgaert, L., Cockmartin, L. et al. (2023). Photon-counting CT allows better visualization of temporal bone structures in comparison with current generation multi-detector CT. *Insights Imaging* 14 (11): https://doi.org/10.1186/s13244-023-01467-w.

18 Macielak, R.J., Benson, J.C., Lane, J.I. et al. (2022). Photon-counting detector CT for temporal bone imaging: up to three times the resolution at half the radiation dose. *Otol. Neurotol.* 43 (10): e1205–e1207.

19 Takahashi, Y., Higaki, F., Sugaya, A. et al. (2023). Evaluation of the ear ossicles with photon-counting detector CT. *Jpn. J. Radiol.* 42: 158–164.

20 Sakaida, H., Ichikawa, Y., Yamazaki, A. et al. (2024). Ultra-high spatial resolution images of the temporal bone obtained with a newly released photon-counting detector computed tomography. *Ear Nose Throat J..*

21 Doyle, N.S., Benson, J.C., Carr, C.M. et al. (2023). Photon counting versus energy-integrated detector CT in detection of superior semicircular canal dehiscence. *Clin. Neuroradiol.* 6: 251–255.

22 Radiology Cafe (2025). Anatomy and pathologies of the abdomen. https://www.radiologycafe.com/radiology-basics/abdomen/abdomen-anatomy/ Accessed February 2025.

23 Pourmorteza, A., Symons, R., Sandfort, V. et al. (2016). Abdominal Imaging with Contrast-enhanced Photon-counting CT: First Human Experience. *Radiology* 279 (1): 239–245. https://doi.org/10.1148/radiol.2016152601.

24 Schwartz, F.R., Samei, E., and Marin, D. (2023). Exploiting the potential of photon-counting CT in abdominal imaging. *Investig. Radiol.* 58 (7): 488–498. https://doi.org/10.1097/RLI.0000000000000949.

25 Graafen, D., Müller, L., Halfmann, M. et al. (2022). Photon-counting detector CT improves quality of arterial phase abdominal scans: A head-to-head comparison with energy-integrating CT. *Eur. J. Radiol.* 156: 110514.

26 Benson, J.C., Campeau, N.G., Diehn, F.E. et al. (2024). Photon-counting ct in the head and neck: current applications and future prospects. *Am. J. Neuroradiol.* https://doi.org/10.3174/ajnr.A8265.

27 Sendić, G. (2025). Musculoskeletal system: anatomy and functions. https://www.kenhub.com/en/library/anatomy/the-musculoskeletal-system (accessed February 2025).

28 Mourad, C., Gallego Manzano, L., Viry, A. et al. (2024). Chances and challenges of photon-counting CT in musculoskeletal imaging. *Skeletal Radiol.* 53: 1889–1902. https://doi.org/10.1007/s00256-024-04622-6.

29 Grunz, J.-P. and MD; Huflage, Henner MD. (2025). Photon-counting detector CT applications in musculoskeletal radiology. *Investig. Radiol.* 60 (3): 198–204. https://doi.org/10.1097/RLI.0000000000001108.

30 Bette, S., Risch, F., Becker, J. et al. (2025). Photon-counting detector CT – first experiences in the field of musculoskeletal radiology. *Fortschr. Röntgenstr.* 197: 34.

31 Grunz, J.P. and Huflage, H. (2024). Photon-counting computed tomography: experience in musculoskeletal imaging. *Korean J. Radiol.* 25 (7): 662–672. https://doi.org/10.3348/kjr.2024.0096.

32 Baffour, F.I., Glazebrook, K.N., Ferrero, A. et al. (2023). Photon-counting detector CT for musculoskeletal imaging: a clinical perspective. *AJR* 220 (4): 551–561. https://doi.org/10.2214/AJR.22.28418.

33 Eibschutz, L.S., Matcuk, G., Chiu, M.K.-J. et al. (2024). Updates on the applications of spectral computed tomography for musculoskeletal imaging. *Diagnostics.* 14 (7): 732. https://doi.org/10.3390/diagnostics14070732.

34 Sharma, S.P., Lemmens, M.J.D.K., Smulders, M.W. et al. (2024). Photon-counting detector computed tomography in cardiac imaging. *Neth. Hear. J.* 32: 405–416. https://doi.org/10.1007/s12471-024-01904-5.

35 Meloni, A., Cademartiri, F., Positano, V. et al. (2023). Cardiovascular applications of photon-counting CT technology: a revolutionary new diagnostic step. *J. Cardiovasc. Dev. Dis.* 10 (9): 363. https://doi.org/10.3390/jcdd10090363.

36 Lacaita, P.G., Luger, A., Troger, F. et al. (2024). Photon-counting detector computed tomography (PCD-CT): a new era for cardiovascular imaging? Current status and future outlooks. *J. Cardiovasc. Dev. Dis.* 11 (4): 127. https://doi.org/10.3390/jcdd11040127.

37 Flohr, T., Schmidt, B., Ulzheimer, S., and Alkadhi, H. (2023). Cardiac imaging with photon counting CT. *Br. J. Radiol.* 96 (1152): 20230407. https://doi.org/10.1259/bjr.20230407.

38 Meloni, A., Maffei, E., Positano, V. et al. (2024). Technical principles, benefits, challenges, and applications of photon counting computed tomography in coronary imaging: a narrative review. *Cardiovasc. Diagn. Ther.* 14 (4): 698–724. https://doi.org/10.21037/cdt-24-52.

Index

Rad Tech's Guide to Photon Counting Computed Tomography,
First Edition. Euclid Seeram.
© 2025 John Wiley & Sons, Inc. Published 2025 by John Wiley & Sons, Inc.

Printed and bound by CPI Group (UK) Ltd, Croydon, CR0 4YY

07/07/2026

14916214-0001